Normal Development of Functional Motor Skills

The First Year of Life

Rona Alexander, Ph.D., CCC-SP
Regi Boehme, OTR
Barbara Cupps, PT

Illustrations by John Boehme

HAMMILL INSTITUTE ON DISABILITIES
8700 SHOAL CREEK BOULEVARD
AUSTIN, TEXAS 78757-6897
512/451-3521 FAX 512/451-3728

Hammill Institute on Disabilities
8700 Shoal Creek Boulevard
Austin, Texas 78757-6897
512/451-3521   Fax 512/451-3728

■ About the Authors

Rona Alexander, Ph.D., CCC-SP, is a speech-language pathologist specializing in assessment and treatment of oral-motor and respiratory-phonatory-sound production functioning in infants and children with neuromotor involvement. She maintains a private practice, is a part-time staff member at the Children's Hospital of Wisconsin in Milwaukee, and conducts workshops on oral-motor and respiratory-phonatory development, assessment, and treatment. She is a qualified speech instructor in Neuro-Developmental Treatment.

Although *Normal Development of Functional Motor Skills* is Rona's first book for Therapy Skill Builders, she has contributed chapters on oral-motor/feeding and respiratory-phonatory function to numerous publications.

After receiving an A.B. degree in speech pathology and audiology from Indiana University, Rona continued in the speech pathology field to receive an M.A. degree from New York University and a Ph.D. degree from the University of Illinois at Urbana-Champaign. She is a member of NDTA, AACPDM, and ASHA. In 1990 she received the Outstanding Clinical Achievement Award from the Wisconsin Speech-Language-Hearing Association.

Regi Boehme, OTR/L, has been involved with the assessment and treatment of neurologically challenged children and adults for more than 25 years. She owns and operates a Milwaukee-based treatment clinic and a treatment center near Billings, Montana, providing assessment and treatment for pediatric and adult patients from around the world. She provides international clinical training programs for physical, occupational, and speech therapists.

Normal Development of Functional Motor Skills is Regi's second publication for Therapy Skill Builders, who is also a distributor for many of her clinical practice manuals. Her first book, *Improving Upper Body Control,* concerns upper extremity assessment and treatment of patients with neurological challenges.

Regi received a B.S. degree in occupational therapy from Western Michigan University. She is a registered Occupational Therapist with AOTA and is licensed in both Wisconsin and Montana. She has been a certified NDT Occupational Therapy Instructor since 1979.

Barbara Cupps, PT, is a physical therapist with her own private practice in Milwaukee. She is a coordinator instructor of basic and advanced courses in pediatric Neuro-Developmental Treatment and gives numerous seminars and short courses pertaining to assessment and treatment of children who have central nervous system dysfunction.

Normal Development of Functional Motor Skills is Barbara's first publication with Therapy Skill Builders. After receiving a B.S. degree in physical therapy from Marquette University, Barbara continued her education with courses in Neuro-Developmental Treatment as well as other treatment approaches. She is a member of APTA and NDTA.

■ About the Illustrator

John Boehme graduated from St. Norberts College in Wisconsin with a B.S. degree in psychology. His avocation of stained glass designing has led to his "love of line" that is expressed in his illustrations. He is the executive director of Boehme Workshops, which offer state-of-the-art continuing education opportunities for individuals involved in the care of children with neurological dysfunction.

■ Preface

The material in this text is based on our observations of normally developing infants between birth and twelve months of age. We first observed and photographed babies in 1981. From that experience, we created developmental guidelines, which were used in assessment and treatment planning and shared with students in our workshops. In 1990-91, we observed, photographed, and studied a second group of normally developing babies in preparation for this text.

The purpose of this work is to assist clinicians, teachers, and other pediatric team members in their understanding of how children develop specific functional skills during the first twelve months of life. Such information can be a useful tool in the treatment planning process for children with neurological involvement and developmental disabilities. It can also be used as a guideline for assessing functional motor levels in children.

During our observations of infants, we were consistently amazed by the differences in when and how they developed functional motor skills. In terms of assessment and treatment, this points out our need to expect and respond to the variety of movement patterns that children develop in their quest for independence.

■ Acknowledgments

The authors thank the following individuals for their assistance in the development and completion of this book:

The babies and their families for allowing us to study and photograph them and generally disrupt their lives.

Our families and friends for their patience, endurance, and flexibility.

Chris Damask Beesley for typing this manuscript.

Mary Ellen Boehme for editing.

Berta Bobath, Lois Bly, and Helen Mueller for their contributions to our learning.

Contents

Chapter 1

Concepts Underlying the Development of Movement

Traditional studies of normal motor development have revolved around models of reflexes and neural maturation. However, neither adequately addresses the variety and complexity of movement. Knowledge of the nervous system has been rapidly expanding while knowledge of the qualitative and quantitative aspects of movement has remained largely subjective. Recent technological advances have now resulted in greater analysis of the kinematic and muscle activity factors involved in movement (Kamm et al. 1990). Results indicate that neural maturation alone does not dictate the process of motor development, but that many other factors also influence movement. Some of these concepts are presented in this chapter as a framework for understanding the process of motor development.

■ Motor Control

The science of motor control evolved in the 1980s to encompass a number of different fields, including neuroscience, psychology, and rehabilitation. Motor learning, the process of acquiring motor control, is an integral part of this relatively new science. Controversy exists and several models of motor control have been proposed. It is beyond the scope of this book to explore these theories; however, some elements appear to be generally accepted and provide a basis for understanding the process by which a baby develops motor skills in the first year of life.

Two types of mechanisms that control the execution of a movement have been described. A feedback or closed-loop type mechanism is one in which sensory information initiates and/or plays a direct role in the coordination of the movement.

This type of mechanism is used for initial acquisition of a skill, especially those which involve complex and discrete movements. The development of skills which involve eye-hand coordination utilizes this type of mechanism. The feedforward or open-loop mechanism may use sensory information prior to the movement and for evaluation after the movement, but sensory input does not change motor output during execution. This type of mechanism is used in rapid movements and in well-learned movements (Giuliani 1991).

Both mechanisms are used in motor control. During the first year of life, the baby often performs new skills slowly and deliberately, using more feedback processes. With practice the skill can be performed without sensory information, using a feedforward mode of execution.

One theory of motor control explains the execution of movement through motor programs, or abstract codes stored in the central nervous system. Some of these programs are innate, such as breathing and kicking, but most are learned. There appears to be an organization of these programs according to the general class of the movement pattern involved; for example, reach. Each program has invariant features that remain constant and variant features that adapt to the specific task at hand (Giuliani 1991). Invariant features include the order of events, timing, and relative force. Other aspects of the movement pattern can vary, such as the overall duration, intensity of muscle contraction, and even the specific muscles and joints used for the activity (Light 1991).

A dynamic systems approach provides a more holistic approach to motor control. This theory suggests that control of movement is the result of many systems working together dynamically. These systems follow basic rules of physics and nature and relate to each other in a cooperative manner. Coordination of movement is affected by many factors including arousal or motivation, neuromuscular activity, musculoskeletal properties, cardiopulmonary function, and environmental factors. A dynamic systems model implies that no one factor (arousal, neuromuscular, sensory) has greater influence than the others, but that all subsystems interact in such a way that a motor behavior emerges that is not specific to any one of the subsystems. This means the system is self-organizing, which is a feature of complex dynamic or nonlinear systems. In a self-organizing system, preferred patterns of behavior develop. Although functional skills can be achieved with a wide variety of possible combinations of factors, the patterns that reflect the most efficient subsystem interaction and that require the least amount of energy are utilized.

The complexity of dynamic systems implies that there are many elements that can vary or change. Bernstein calls these elements degrees of freedom, in reference to neuromotor functioning (Giuliani 1991). This is a more global definition than the biomechanical degrees of freedom involving axes and planes of motion and includes neuromotor as well as musculoskeletal components. The grouping of muscles into patterns of coordination or synergies is one way in which the many degrees of freedom can be constrained. The concept of central programs for the execution of movements also decreases the degrees of freedom (Atwater 1991).

The dynamic pattern theory is another way of explaining how degrees of freedom can be constrained in a complex system. This theory suggests that principles of pattern organization transcend specific structures. It surmises that the neural network provides a supporting framework for movement but does not dictate the pattern (Scholz 1990). Preferred patterns of movement exist but are reorganized or altered when demands on the system dictate a change. Movement patterns are reorganized through control parameters, those variables that provide a condition for a pattern change. These parameters do not dictate what change will occur, but when they reach a critical value, they act as an agent for reorganization of the motor pattern (Heriza 1991). Examples of possible control parameters include arousal, velocity, loading, weight shift (change in center of gravity), and limb stiffness. There are different control parameters for different movement patterns and probably many control parameters for each intrinsic movement pattern.

The transition from one preferred pattern of coordination to another is called a phase shift. During this phase shift the system is in a state of instability until a new preferred pattern is established. While pattern changes occur as part of daily functioning (changing from walking to running), they also occur during the development of motor skills. Many such changes are seen during the first year of life.

■ Postural Control

Postural control provides a background for maintaining a posture against gravity while helping to stabilize forces that result from movement. Posture is the result of many sensory inputs and various control mechanisms. The Bobaths (1964) stated that postural control is a function of the postural reflex mechanism based on the neurophysiology of the time. They believed that postural reactions were responsible for man's ability to get up and stay upright against gravity and at the same time to be mobile.

Although current neurophysiology does not view posture under the control of a "reflex mechanism," evidence is strong that posture and movement are controlled by independent processes and that they are coordinated for the performance of functional skills.

Postural sets or synergies automatically prepare for a functional skilled movement and support it throughout its duration. Frank and Earl (1990) discuss three types of postural control strategies that have been identified for efficient and safe movements. One strategy is postural preparations, a feedforward-type activity that increases stability before the onset of the movement. This may include changing the base of support (for example, widening the stance to lift a heavy load, holding a railing to ascend stairs) and stiffening joints through muscle cocontraction.

A second type of postural adjustment involves changes immediately prior to and during the execution of a movement. These postural accompaniments serve to maintain the center of gravity, to control the displacement of it during movement, or to position it over a new base of support. An anticipatory effect of the movement on posture is required and a feedforward system of control is utilized to activate postural adjustments simultaneously with the movement.

Until recent years the most widely studied type of postural response has been postural reactions. These are responses to unexpected changes in the center of gravity and are controlled by a feedback-type mechanism. Sensory receptors (vestibular, ocular, proprioceptive) detect a loss of balance and trigger a response specific to the direction, amount, and speed of weight shift. These reactions are not always successful in maintaining the center of gravity over the base of support, and falling may result. These reactions have been classified as righting reactions, protective extension, and equilibrium reactions.

At the time of a movement, the most appropriate strategy for postural control is selected, dependent on the internal and external parameters. Activation of certain synergistic muscles is sometimes sufficient to control a posture during movement without a displacement in the center of gravity. This may be especially true during fine motor activities. However, much of our skilled movement requires some degree of weight shift, subtle in some instances and obvious in others. The displacement of the center of gravity is controlled by somewhat predictable patterns depending on the direction, amount, and speed of the weight shift, similar to what occurs in postural reactions. The similarity between patterns of postural accompaniments and postural reactions may indicate that prestructured postural synergies exist that simplify the control of posture (Frank and Earl 1990). This would make coordination of posture with movement easier, given the complexity and almost infinite number of movement patterns available.

For example, if a person is seated on a tilt board and the board is moved so the person's center of gravity moves forward, a postural reaction occurs. This results in the head, neck, trunk, and hip moving toward extension (optical righting, equilibrium). A seated person who reaches forward and upward actively shifts the center of gravity anteriorly, and similar muscle activation patterns are utilized. When the arm is elevated without a weightshift forward, the extensors still contract to stabilize the head and trunk as the arm moves upward.

In addition to postural activity in regard to movement, postural tone has been viewed as part of postural control. The Bobaths (1964) stated that normal tone is sufficiently high to maintain a posture against gravity yet low enough to be mobile. Although they used the term muscle tone interchangeably with postural tone, they discussed that tone involved the musculature of the entire body and was automatically coordinated in definite patterns (Bobath and Bobath 1959). Postural tone is a global phenomenon that may include muscle tone (intrinsic properties and neural activation of a specific muscle). Recently the term stiffness has been used to describe a characteristic of the intrinsic properties of muscles in regard to flexibility. This is only one aspect of muscle tone that may contribute to postural tone.

Because external forces act on the body, there needs to be a mechanism that stabilizes postures independent of movement. Variations are seen from one individual to another (that is, some hold erect postures easily and others tend to slouch or lean). Although, optimally, much of the stability to hold postures results from structural stability of the musculoskeletal system, it alone is not sufficient. Maintaining posture is a multiple system process including a muscular activity that can be considered to be one aspect of postural tone. This control acts in a direction opposite to the external force and requires a supporting surface to work against. For example, to maintain an erect posture in sitting, pelvic girdle activity can generate a force against the seat. Spinal muscles activate progressively upward, and a stable and efficient alignment is achieved.

The postural control system develops from birth and continues throughout life. Postural responses appear to develop in a cephalocaudal direction, beginning at the head and neck and progressively emerging in the trunk and lower extremities. Postural synergies that accompany movement develop and become consistent with practice, but the specific pattern varies from one individual to another. These synergies continually develop through adulthood whenever new motor skills are learned.

During the process of developing motor skills, a baby uses certain positions that provide mechanical stability when postural control is immature. For example, in prone, the hip flexion/abduction/external rotation posture of a three-month-old baby stabilizes the lower body as the baby lifts the head. By five months, hip extensor activity is evident, providing dynamic rather than mechanical stability. According to the dynamic pattern theory, this demonstrates a phase shift in the pattern of lifting the upper body in prone. The system may be in a more unstable state at this time and one or more control parameters may be responsible for the system reorganizing. Possibilities include the increased mobility of the spine and hip joints, muscle strength, and motivation.

Another method for providing stability for development of movement is to limit the degrees of freedom by "fixing" or holding parts of the body through muscle contraction (Bly 1991). For example, shoulder elevation is utilized by the infant to stabilize and support the head. In another example, the infant utilizes cocontraction of agonist and antagonist around the ankle joint for optimal stability in early independent standing and walking. However, as postural organization develops, the cocontraction is replaced by synergistic patterns that are more efficient. These strategies are a common way of dealing with instability when postural control is developing.

■ Musculoskeletal System

The development of functional motor skills is clearly dependent on the development of the musculoskeletal system. The many subsystems included in this area involve not only bone and muscle, but also neuromuscular connections, joints, and soft tissue such as tendons, ligaments, and other fascia. Although structurally these elements develop in utero, they undergo change throughout life dependent on their function within the system as well as on the functioning of other systems.

Walker (1991) states that many investigators believe all muscle fibers are present in early infancy and that major change occurs in the size of the muscle fibers. Functional demands placed on the system influence the chemical processes of muscle function and the size of the muscle fibers. For example, the need for adequate respiration accounts for the relatively large muscle fibers of the diaphragm at birth. They are twice the size of the fibers of the intercostals or limb musculature (Walker 1991). Growth and the development of antigravity movement require increased muscle strength, placing a great demand on muscle fibers to hypertrophy in the first year of life.

The relationship between growth and muscle strength affects the development of posture and movement. Studies have suggested that the disappearance of automatic stepping in infancy is the result of weight gain without a corresponding increase in muscle strength (Kamm et al. 1990). For a few months, the infant is too weak to step. The assumption can be made that some motor skills emerge when sufficient muscle strength has developed in relation to body mass. In addition to strength, the baby requires increased levels of endurance that are dependent on the functions of the cardiovascular, pulmonary, and metabolic systems. The baby's relentless repetition of movement patterns is important for muscular development, strength, and endurance as well as for motor learning.

Skeletal components change significantly during growth and development and affect posture and movement. Shaping of bones occurs at least partially in response to the forces exerted on them. Although bone remodeling occurs throughout life, the infant has a yearly rate ten times higher than the adult. By age two all primary bone has undergone some remodeling (Walker 1991). The torsion changes that occur in the long bones of the leg demonstrate the effect of remodeling on posture. Complex relationships exist between hip joint rotation and bony torsion of the femur and tibia that account for the one-year-old child standing and walking with legs turned out. They also account for the two- or three-year-old child appearing to stand with genu valgus (knock-knee), and the adult standing with the mature biomechanical alignment of the lower extremities.

The musculoskeletal system is an "overcomplete" system. It provides movement in many directions and has more muscles than are required for functional movement. Keshner (1990) states that such a complex system allows a single movement pattern to be generated by multiple sensory inputs and a variety of muscle activation patterns. Stability of a system with many degrees of freedom is extremely complex and requires a combination of control mechanisms including mechanical, feedforward, and feedback types. This stability develops individually based on experience and is an integral part of motor learning.

The compact nature of the full-term newborn provides mechanical stability to the musculoskeletal system. Limited range of motion in many joints and closely packed soft tissue elements help provide stability until other mechanisms are more developed. However, elongation of muscle and fascia and joint capsule flexibility needs to occur for the development of functional motor skills. A balance of mobility and stability is required for efficient and coordinated movement.

Postural stability is achieved in part through biomechanical alignment, which also contributes to effective muscle action. In upright posture, optimal alignment of the joints provides stability through the joint configurations and ligamentous structures, minimizing the amount of muscle activity required (figure 1.1). If malalignment is present, greater muscle activity or compensatory alignments of other joints are required. Postural patterns develop in conjunction with skeletal alignment. For example, the toddler stands with increased hip flexion/external rotation and, therefore, requires greater thoraco-lumbar extension to maintain the head and trunk upright.

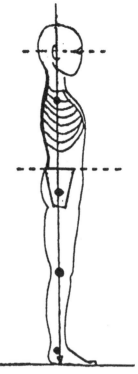

FIGURE 1.1

The biomechanics of a moving body part are affected by both internal and external forces. Gravity is a critical external force acting on the musculoskeletal system to which the central nervous system must accommodate both in posture and movement. Internal forces are generated by the stiffness of adjoining parts and their articulations. In addition, one body segment can exert a force on other body segments. For example, when the baby extends a leg during kicking, a force is generated that tends to pull the pelvis along with the femur. This results in extension of the lumbar spine. The biomechanics during a movement are extremely complex as these combined forces are not constant, but change with speed, intensity, and direction of the movement in space. The development of coordinated movement demands the cooperation of many systems to accommodate these factors.

■ Sensory Systems

The role of the sensory systems in motor control is crucial and incredibly complex. The central nervous system continuously receives sensory input, filters the information, disregards some sensations, and processes others. Sensory input can increase or decrease arousal states and be the motivating force to initiate motor activity. The baby utilizes all aspects of the sensory system to stimulate and reinforce motor behavior. For example, vision is the motivational focus for the development of head control. The auditory channel stimulates vision, hand, and cognitive development. The baby is also motivated to repeat movements for the pleasure that kinesthetic and vestibular sensations provide.

Sensory systems guide and organize motor activity. In feedback modes of motor control, sensory information is used to detect and correct errors in the accuracy of a movement. During the first year of life, the baby learns many motor skills through the information provided by the tactile, kinesthetic, and vestibular systems in response to visual and auditory input. Sensory input is utilized to evaluate motor performance in feedforward-type movements. This may result in a new preferred pattern of coordination or in a greater repertoire of dynamic patterns to accommodate specific conditions of a motor task.

■ Motor Learning

Motor learning can be studied from many aspects. Much current literature contains information regarding acquisition of new motor skills by an adult. Theories that relate to practice methods and feedback strategies have become very sophisticated. However, the process by which a baby learns motor skills is not well documented.

The traditional models of neural maturation and hierarchy control of the central nervous system are no longer adequate. The concepts of a dynamic systems approach to motor control need to be integrated into our understanding of motor development. Heriza (1991) has expanded the dynamic systems approach to include developmental factors.

A schema for the coordination of posture and movement has been presented by Frank and Earl (1990). This model can be used to illustrate some principles of motor learning as well as motor performance (figure 1.2).

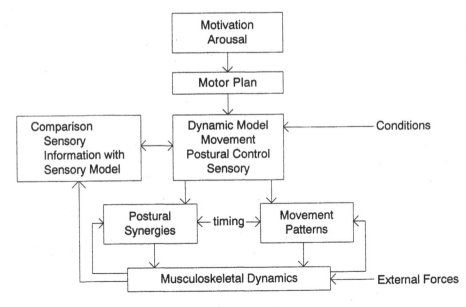

FIGURE 1.2. Adapted from Frank and Earl 1990.

The concepts of arousal states and motivation are extremely important for motor activity and motor learning. The model in figure 1.2 demonstrates that motivation precedes and is critical for movement. The arousal state of the infant is important in the overall development. The infant must be sufficiently aroused to be motivated to attend, move, and explore the environment. On the other hand, if overaroused, the infant either is irritable or falls asleep. With an appropriate level of arousal comes the baby's curiosity about the world, a strong desire to gain control of the body, and the pleasure of repeating a skill until it becomes efficient and automatic.

The schema presented in figure 1.2 includes a motor plan and a dynamic model for execution of a movement. Frank and Earl (1990) suggest that motor plans are translated into movement parameters through a model of body dynamics. This model develops through repetition of movements and the sensory feedback that accompanies those movements. The dynamic model includes both the focal movements and the postural synergies as well as the timing between them. A sensory model of the dynamics also is included. Sensory information can be utilized to determine if the goal of the movement is achieved or if the result is different from what was expected. The dynamic model can then be altered. In the infant, the model of body dynamics is not well developed and postural responses are absent or inadequate. As the baby performs motor patterns, the dynamic model evolves as a result of many interacting systems, and skill development occurs.

When the system determines that a motor plan is to be executed, it scans its repertoire for the specific dynamic model needed to perform the desired activity. It takes into account the general category of the task and the specific conditions at the time. These may include position in space, base of support, load, and end goal. For example, the desire to kick a ball can trigger a motor plan. The conditions could be running while kicking a soccer ball into a goal. A different set of conditions exists when a child stands and kicks a beach ball across the sand. An important part of motor development includes expanding the different sets of conditions so that movement becomes skilled and functional.

■ Summary

Many concepts underlie the development of movement, some of which have been discussed in this chapter. Although new theories of motor control are still evolving, they can provide a framework for understanding the process by which babies acquire motor skills. The dynamic systems approach to motor behavior suggests that skills emerge as the result of many systems and subsystems interacting in a cooperative manner. Within this framework, motor development progresses through many circular loops and mechanisms of control (Atwater 1991). Development is not a linear process, but rather has phases of intense and overlapping motor activity. When motor skills emerge in one area, other functions may remain constant or even regress. For example, a baby that begins to walk independently often produces fewer sounds in the upright position.

Past knowledge of the developmental process can be incorporated into the theories of motor control, bringing us to a new level of understanding. All aspects of a child's life, including environmental interaction, play a role in motor skill acquisition.

Similarly, motor development can impact on social, emotional, and cognitive development. Therefore, we should not be surprised or confused when children develop motor skills at different rates with varying patterns of postural control and movement. The following chapters contain examples of how and when babies perform motor activities in different functional areas. The material should not be viewed as a rigid timetable or a strict model of motor behavior.

■ References

Atwater, S. 1991. Should the normal motor developmental sequence be used as a theoretical model in pediatric physical therapy? In *Contemporary management of motor control problems: Proceedings of the II STEP conference*, edited by M. Lister, 89-93. Alexandria, VA: Foundation for Physical Therapy.

Bly, L. 1991. A historical and current view of the basis of NDT. *Pediatric Physical Therapy* 3:131-35.

Bobath, K., and B. Bobath. 1964. The facilitation of normal postural reactions and movements in the treatment of cerebral palsy. *Physiotherapy* 50(8):246-62.

_____. 1959. The neuropathology of cerebral palsy and its importance in treatment and diagnosis. *Cerebral Palsy Bulletin* 1(8):13-33.

Frank, J., and M. Earl. 1990. Coordination of posture and movement. *Physical Therapy* 70:855-63.

Giuliani, C. 1991. Theories of motor control: New concepts for physical therapy. In *Contemporary management of motor control problems: Proceedings of the II STEP conference*, edited by M. Lister, 29-35. Alexandria, VA: Foundation for Physical Therapy.

Heriza, C. 1991. Motor development: Traditional and contemporary theories. In *Contemporary management of motor control problems: Proceedings of the II STEP conference*, edited by M. Lister, 99-126. Alexandria, VA: Foundation for Physical Therapy.

Kamm, K., E. Thelen, and J. Jensen. 1990. A dynamic systems approach to motor development. *Physical Therapy* 70:763-75.

Keshner, E. 1990. Controlling stability of a complex movement system. *Physical Therapy* 70:844-54.

Light, K. 1991. Unpublished notes from lecture.

Scholz, J. 1990. Dynamic pattern theory—some implications for therapeutics. *Physical Therapy* 70:827-43.

Walker, J. 1991. Musculoskeletal development: A review. *Physical Therapy* 71:878-89.

Chapter 2

Newborn

■ Postural Control

The ability to maintain postures and stabilize movements in a gravity dependent environment develops over time. However, an infant is born with mechanisms that provide some control in the early months. One of these mechanisms creates an imbalance between flexor and extensor muscle tone so that flexor tone dominates, contributing to the overall flexed posture of the newborn infant. The concept of "muscle tone" has not been well defined, but appears to be relative to intrinsic properties of muscle as well as neural activity that produces muscle contraction. Although the origin of the newborn's tone is not known, it is well demonstrated in the flexor recoil of the limbs. When you stretch out the arm or leg, it actively returns to a flexed position. Sometimes referred to as "physiological flexion," this tone is different from anti-gravity flexor control that develops in postural activity (Bly 1983); yet it does tend to hold the baby compact and provide a sufficient base of stability for random movements to occur.

Although not complete, some righting reactions are present at birth. Rotation of the head stimulates proprioceptors in the neck, resulting in the body rotating to follow the head (neck righting). Labyrinthine righting is just beginning and can be observed in prone when the infant slightly lifts and turns the head. It is also seen in a semi-reclined supine position when the infant attempts to lift the head. As the infant is pulled to a sitting position, some activation of the flexors may be felt; however, the head lags behind the shoulders (figure 2.1). When the newborn is placed upright on the feet, the primary standing reaction can be elicited with the knees, hips and spine progressively extending

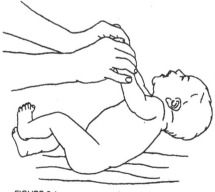

FIGURE 2.1

11

upward (figure 2.2). These initial postural reactions further develop in the next six months. Similar co-ordinative patterns develop to accompany movement and are adapted for specific functional activities throughout life.

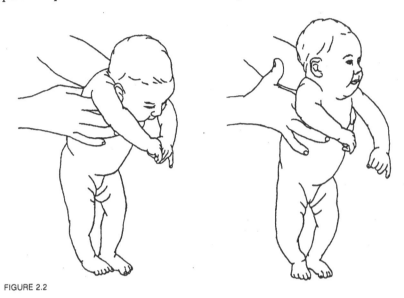

FIGURE 2.2

■ Gross Motor Development

Anatomical/Structural Characteristics

Anatomical differences between the newborn and the adult impact on the development of posture and movement. One variable is the relative size of one body part to another. For example, compared to the adult, the newborn's head is proportionally larger than the rest of the body and the lower extremities are short in comparison to the upper limbs and torso. Another variable is the contour of bony structures. Most bones have not completely ossified at birth, rather some areas are cartilaginous. Bony shaping occurs during growth, at least partially due to the mechanical forces exerted on the skeleton. These forces may be internal, including the forces generated by tension of tendons and ligaments and by muscle contraction. There are also external forces, such as gravity and the pressure exerted by a supporting surface.

The vertebral column exemplifies a change in skeletal contour during growth. In the newborn, the spine is relatively straight except for two flexion curves. One is a shallow thoracic curve with its apex located at approximately the T-4 to T-6 level, gently sloping to vertical by the level of C-7. The other is the flexed sacral-coccygeal area (figure 2.3). Secondary curves into extension develop in the cervical and lumbar areas and, with continued changes in these primary curves, form the "S-shaped" adult spine. In the newborn, the spinous processes of the vertebrae are nearly horizontal rather than curved downward as in the adult.

Another example of bony shaping occurs in the femur. The femoral angle, or angle of inclination, which is formed by the neck and shaft of the femur, changes from 150 degrees at birth to 125 degrees in the adult (Norkin and Levangie 1983). Therefore, the femur is relatively more adducted, narrowing the base of support for a more efficient weight shift in walking (figure 2.4). Dynamic forces exerted by muscle activity around the hip play a role in effecting this change; elongation of the iliopsoas muscle group also is important. In addition, an internal torsion of the long axis or shaft of the femur gradually decreases from an average of 30 degrees at birth to approximately 10 degrees by adulthood.

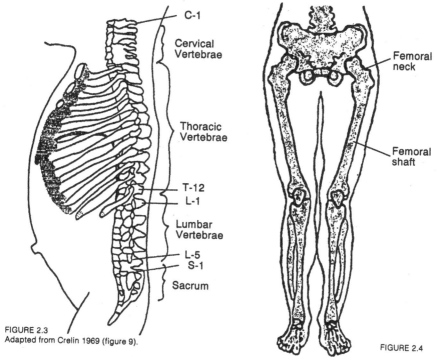

FIGURE 2.3
Adapted from Crelin 1969 (figure 9).

FIGURE 2.4

Range of Motion

Range of motion is limited in many joints of the full-term newborn. Although the reasons are not clearly understood, flexor tone and the limited space in utero during the last weeks of pregnancy probably contribute to soft tissue and capsular inflexibility. In the spine, extension as well as lateral and rotational ranges of motion are limited. However, spinal mobility increases dramatically in the first six months of life and directly influences shoulder and pelvic girdle motion.

Lower extremity mobility is also limited in the newborn. Hip range is limited in extension, abduction, and internal rotation, at least partially due to the shortened iliopsoas muscles that flex, abduct, and externally rotate the hip. As a result of both capsular tightness and limited hamstring length, the knees of many newborns cannot be completely extended. Increased mobility is seen only in the ankles where dorsiflexion is excessive while plantar flexion is limited.

Functional range of motion depends on soft tissue and skeletal considerations as well as on muscle activity. These factors change in growth and development, allowing greater mobility, stability, and efficiency of posture and movement.

Posture and Movement

At rest, the full-term newborn infant demonstrates a flexed posture, the degree of flexion dependent on individual passive tone, range of motion, and position in space. The head is rarely in midline but rather slightly rotated. The spine tends to be flexed in the thoracic area. The hips are flexed, adducted, and externally rotated. The knees are flexed, and the feet are dorsiflexed.

In prone, the baby's pelvis is raised off the surface by the excessive hip flexion (figure 2.5), causing the center of gravity to be more cephalic so much of the body weight is transferred to the head and shoulders. This makes movement of the head and arms in prone very difficult. The baby can lift the head and turn it slightly in an attempt to maintain an open airway for breathing. Random movements are not as frequent as in supine. The baby may stretch one or both legs into extension; however, the legs quickly return to flexion. Some newborns do not like prone and fuss and squirm when placed in this position.

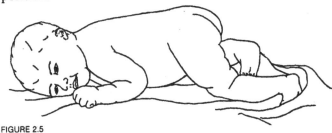

FIGURE 2.5

Posture is less flexed in supine as gravity tends to favor extension (figure 2.6). The shoulders are less protracted than in prone, and the arms are more abducted. The hips are less flexed/adducted and may be more externally rotated, especially in an infant with a lower tone base. More movement is available in this position; however, babies are not as stable as in prone and may startle with their own random movements, even awakening from sleep. Swaddling minimizes this by providing external stability until there is sufficient maturation of postural control. The infant may turn the head, rhythmically move one or both arms, one or both legs, one arm and a leg on the same or opposite sides, or all four limbs. The infant may stretch into asymmetrical extension, resulting in rotation of the spine, or may pull into a total flexion pattern. Some active newborn infants may actually "roll over" in this manner.

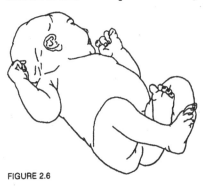

FIGURE 2.6

Sidelying is a position often recommended for newborns. When swaddled in a blanket, they can be in a flexed posture, have an open airway, and, consequently, are less likely to choke. Some movements in a small controlled range are available to them, especially hand-to-hand and hand-to-mouth activities.

When newborn infants are placed in sitting, physiological flexion, joint immobility, and decreased flexibility of soft tissue allow them to maintain the position briefly, keeping them from flopping like a rag doll. The pelvis is vertical with weight on the ischial tuberosities, but the spine is flexed with the head forward, causing the center of gravity to be anterior to the hip joint. Consequently, if unsupported, the baby slowly rolls forward to the surface, the center of gravity following the head and shoulders, transferring weight to the upper body. Then, as the pelvis is now unweighted, the infant extends the legs out from under the body, ending up in a prone position.

The automatic stepping reaction is also present in the first few weeks. When the infant is placed on the feet with the center of gravity slightly forward, the legs flex and extend reciprocally. Although similar to the mature pattern of walking, hip flexion is exaggerated in step and the extension is more rapid with the forefoot making the initial contact with the surface. The stance leg does not bear full weight or push against the surface for propulsion; additionally, weightshift and postural control are absent. Automatic stepping appears to be generated at the spinal level and may be the result of a central program of neural control (Myklebust 1990). Maturation of the central nervous system together with other systems results in adaptations of this program for functional walking. Automatic stepping and random kicking also have similar kinematic patterns suggesting that they are isomorphic, or one and the same movement pattern, but differ in their developmental course (Kamm et al. 1990).

Random Movements

A continuation of movements in utero, random movements of the head, spine, and limbs, are present at birth. These movements do not require a specific stimulus and are not well defined, rather there is a great deal of variety and individual differences. One study identified eighty types of movement in the newborn infant (Weggeman et al. 1987), categorizing them into the following six areas:

1. *Progression movements.* Rhythmic alternating flexion/extension movements of one, two, or four limbs in any combination with or without head movement. They resemble the swimming movements of the fetus and may have the same basic pattern as stepping, creeping, climbing, and swimming.

2. *Symmetrical movements.* Total body movements that are executed more slowly than progressive movements. They can be in an extensor pattern (head back, spine arching, extension of the arms with internal rotation and hip/knee/toe extension) or a flexion pattern (head flexed, spine rounded, and elbows/hips/knees flexed). Asymmetry may result in a rotational component in the trunk.

3. *Startle.* Quick brief movements of the head, trunk, and limbs into flexion; the hands are closed.

4. *Asymmetrical tonic neck reflex and moro.* When the baby turns the head to one side, the arm and leg on the skull side may flex. If the infant's random movements cause a too-quick roll to the side from supine, the head may go back, arms abduct, and hands open. Other primitive reflexes could be included in this group as they are sometimes elicited by the infant's own random movements. For example, if the foot touches the side of the cradle in rhythmical kicking, a supporting reaction or a withdrawal movement might occur. None of these reflexes are obligatory, but can interrupt or inhibit other types of movement.

5. *Facial movements.* Include smiles, grimaces, eyelid opening and closing, eye movements, sucking, and tongue movements.

6. *Distal isolated movements.* Spontaneous supination/pronation with wrist and finger movements and extension and abduction of the toes.

The infant's movements tend to be somewhat jerky and tremors may occur, especially in the end ranges of movements as a result of an immature central nervous system. Spinal circuitry demonstrates reciprocal excitation in the newborn infant as reciprocal inhibition has not yet developed. Accordingly, if a stretch is elicited, contractions of agonist and antagonist muscles may occur. This monosynaptic pathway is hyperexcitable in the neonate. Also when a stretch reflex is elicited in distal muscles, EMG activity is recorded in more proximal muscles. The apparent spread from one level of the spinal cord to another is called "reflex irradiation" (Myklebust 1990). These phenomena probably are reflected in the infant's random movements. Although the limbs tend to move in total patterns, spatial and temporal aspects of the joint movements are not always in synchrony.

The infant's random movements tend to vary with position, arousal state, and comfort. Movements tend to increase with stimulation, excitement, discomfort (hunger, cold), and crying. In addition to kinesthetic, tactile, and proprioceptive input, these movements provide a mechanism for increasing passive joint ranges and elongating soft tissue. As a body part moves and approaches the end of its passive range, momentum pulls the adjoining parts into the movement. For example, as the leg extends and reaches maximum range at the hip, the pelvis tips anteriorly and the lumbar spine is extended mechanically. Repetition increases range of motion of the hips and lumbar spine.

■ Fine Motor Development

Anatomical/Structural Characteristics

The shoulder girdle is a floating system with many interrelated parts (figure 2.7). The biomechanical attachment of the whole arm and scapula occur at the acromioclavicular joint. The arm, scapula, and clavicle are attached to the body anteriorly, at the sternoclavicular joint (figure 2.8). The glenoid fossa is small and shallow in comparison to the large head of the humerus, allowing wide ranges of arm motion with little

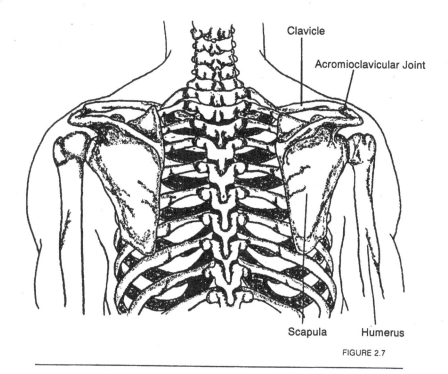

FIGURE 2.7

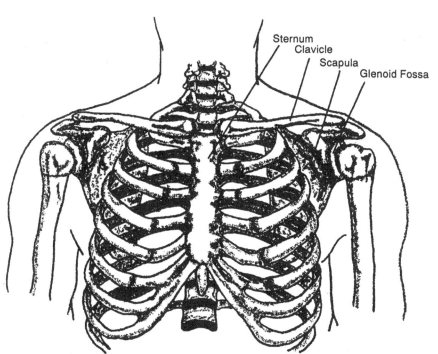

FIGURE 2.8

bony joint stability. The sternum, then, is the only part of the shoulder complex that is well supported biomechanically. Due to the complexity of this system and lack of stable biomechanical support, shoulder girdle control for reach and weight bearing strongly relies on balanced muscle activity.

As in the spine and lower extremities, joint range throughout the shoulder girdle is limited by soft tissue and capsular inflexibility. This results in limited active movements of the upper extremities so that the humerus is rarely elevated above shoulder level and cannot horizontally adduct across the chest. At rest and in prone, the baby's arms are adducted with a forward shoulder position (protraction). The scapulae are elevated and anteriorly tipped. Elbows, wrists, and fingers are flexed. Forearms are pronated. The infant's random movements begin to lengthen soft tissue structures and mobilize joint capsules of the sternum, clavicle, and humerus. Scapulae begin to glide more freely over the rib cage. Prone weight bearing activates the small rotator cuff muscles, creating stability within the glenohumeral joint.

Upper Extremity Development

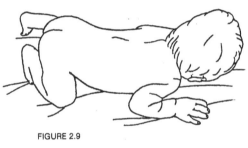

FIGURE 2.9

The upper extremities and head bear the majority of the newborn infant's body weight in prone due to the elevated position of the pelvis (figure 2.9). This weight creates a demand on the shoulders to develop early. As the infant lifts and turns the head, additional weight is transferred to the arms and shoulders. Moreover, as the infant randomly kicks the legs, more body weight and an even greater demand is placed on the upper body. In actuality, the arms and shoulders are receiving a transfer of weight from two directions.

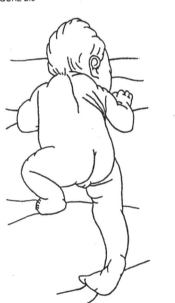

FIGURE 2.10

Initially, the upper extremities passively accept the weight. The glenohumeral joints collapse toward the weight-bearing surface, increasing the forward position of the shoulders (figure 2.10). The elbows are biomechanically raised off the surface, transferring additional body weight onto the forearms, wrists, and radial aspect of the hands. Within approximately 10 to 14 days after birth, the small rotator cuff muscles begin to activate by adducting the humerus into the glenoid fossa. This creates active joint stability, allowing the shoulders to accept the transfer of body weight without collapse. The small rotator cuff muscles provide an important base of stability for random movements, early swiping, and future shoulder girdle development in weight bearing.

The initial forward collapse of the shoulders provides important proprioceptive and kinesthetic information. As the shoulders are forced to move into a greater forward range, the scapulae are mobilized on the rib cage and the humeri are mobilized within their joint structures. The lower trapezius, which will aid with scapular depression, is fully lengthened and stimulated in the process. The flexion and pronation of the wrist and forearm are inhibited, and the muscles are elongated as the weight is transferred to the lower arm.

As the newborn infant concurrently rotates the head and kicks the legs, the upper thoracic spine is mobilized into rotation (see figure 2.10). Motion in this aspect of the spine stimulates medial scapular activity in the first and second month. In addition, this asymmetrical transfer of weight provides each shoulder with contrasting motions. One shoulder moves forward as the other moves posteriorly. This isolated motion prepares the shoulder for specialized control at the five-month level.

In supine, the infant's head, trunk, and scapulae are supported while gravity supplies sufficient force to lengthen the pectoralis major, expanding the upper chest. The combination of gravitational force and the infant's own random movements allow the arms to move away from the body as the baby stretches (figure 2.11). The baby also moves the arms in a somewhat disorganized fashion, using the momentum created through whole body motion. The baby wiggles, flings the arms and legs in all directions, kicks and twitches (Caplan 1971). Full joint range in upper extremity motion is not yet available; consequently the infant rarely is able to move the arm above 90 degrees. The tendency is to move within a horizontal and adduction plane as well as an internal and external rotational plane. As the arm abducts with elbow extension, the hand opens. This "open" orientation of the body may initially frighten or startle the infant to retreat into a fetal position.

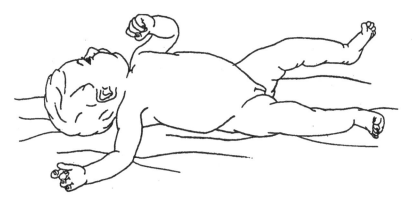

FIGURE 2.11

When newborn infants are placed in sidelying, their arms move toward midline where positional hand-to-hand contact and reflexive hand-to-mouth contact is possible (figure 2.12). The scapulae biomechanically abduct, lengthening medial scapular muscles. Scapular winging is to be expected in this position since newborn infants lack active scapular stability on the rib cage.

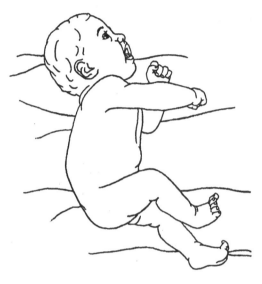

FIGURE 2.12

Hand Development

Infants' hands are generally fisted with the thumb placed inside or outside the palm. The grasp reflex is strong, but the position of the wrist and digits varies in response to the position of the arm. When the arm abducts and the elbow extends, the hand frequently opens (see figure 2.11).

Infants have no specific reach or grasp approach response to stimulus (Erhardt 1982). However, when an object makes contact with the palm, the infant reflexively grasps it. The baby has no voluntary capability to release an object that has been placed in the hand. The object must be forcibly removed or the infant inadvertently drops it as the arm randomly moves away from the body. Newborn infants give no visual attention to their hands.

Visual Development

Newborn infants can see and their world looks brighter than ours with fewer lines and textures (Maurer and Maurer 1988). Initially they are sensitive to light and may keep their eyes closed for a few hours or several days after birth. During these first few days of life, they are unable to visually fixate, but they do have a visual regard for the environment. However, they have no understanding that anything apart from themselves exists (Maurer and Maurer 1988). Their eye movements are random and disorganized.

Within the first week, babies begin to visually fixate with monocular vision (Erhardt 1990). The image from the inactive eye is ignored or suppressed by the central nervous system and they often close the inactive eye. Without this suppression, infants would see double or superimposed images. Thus, they initially learn to control the movements of each eye separately. Infants can follow moving objects in small ranges from the periphery to midline and back. They see moving objects more readily than stationary ones since stationary objects blend or disappear into the background (Jan et al. 1987). Eye movements are not separated from head movements so visual scanning is dependent on the infant's ability to move the head from side to side. When infants visually track, their whole body is in motion. In particular, leg kicking seems to generate the spinal momentum for head turning.

Although visual tracking is easiest in supine where infants can rotate their heads, they are generally more attentive or aroused in a supported upright position. Consequently, they are motivated to develop antigravity head control as an avenue for expanded visual contact with their world.

■ Oral-Motor and Respiratory Development

Anatomical/Structural Characteristics

Oral and pharyngeal mechanisms are involved in many aspects of human function. They are significant parts of the upper respiratory system, the upper digestive system, and the human vocal tract through which phonation and speech are produced. Although the functions of these systems are distinctive, they often overlap, requiring the structures and musculature of the oral and pharyngeal mechanisms to work in a highly organized manner.

The following sections describe the skeletal structures and musculature that compose the oral and pharyngeal mechanisms. These sections are intended as a review to establish an anatomical foundation from which the development of the functional movements of these mechanisms can be better understood. If you require more specific information, resources that focus extensively on the anatomical/structural aspects of the oral and pharyngeal mechanisms of the infant, child, and adult are available. A few resources are Bosma (1986), Crelin (1969, 1973), Netter (1979), and Perkins and Kent (1986).

The oral mechanism. The primary structures that compose the newborn infant's oral mechanism (figures 2.13 and 2.14) include the maxilla (upper jaw), mandible (lower jaw), lips, cheeks, tongue, floor of the mouth, hard palate, soft palate (velum or pharyngeal palate), uvula, and anterior and posterior faucial arches. The oral cavity, or mouth, of the newborn infant is actually the area bounded superiorly by the hard and soft palates, posteriorly by the posterior faucial arch, laterally by the alveolar ridges (alveolar processes or arches) and cheeks, anteriorly by the alveolar ridges and lips, and inferiorly by the tongue and its soft tissue membrane connecting to the mandible. Although the overall size of the newborn's mouth is small in comparison to that of the adult, it is large when viewed in terms of the space it occupies within the infant's face.

The maxilla is actually a paired structure that borders the mouth, nasal cavity, and orbits of the eyes. Its alveolar and palatine processes are of primary significance to the oral cavity. The alveolar processes covered by gum tissue contain dental buds for the deciduous teeth (temporary or primary teeth) as well as buds for the permanent teeth (secondary teeth), which are located above and behind the deciduous teeth.

The palatine processes of the maxilla are continuous posteriorly with the palatine bones, forming the hard or bony palate. At birth the hard palate is short and shallow with only a slight arch and somewhat U-shaped. The oral surface of the hard palate is porous with a series of transverse grooves (rugae) that appear to assist the infant in holding the nipple during breastfeeding or bottledrinking.

Attached to the posterior aspect of the hard palate is the soft palate. It has a prominent median fibromuscular bundle made up of connective tissue and muscles of the uvula. A large portion of the soft palate is composed of musculature that elevates it (levator veli palatini), lowers it (palatophyarngeus and palatoglossus), or stretches it and makes it taut (tensor veli palatini) after growth and musculature activity changes begin at four to six months of age. The palatoglossus muscle, which inserts into the tongue, and the palatopharyngeus muscle, which inserts into the pharyngeal wall, form the anterior and posterior faucial arches, respectively, at the posterior border of the oral cavity. At the end of the median fibromuscular bundle is the soft, flexible uvula that, in the newborn infant, is in approximation with the tip of the epiglottis.

The infant's mandible or jaw is actually composed of a pair of bones that are joined by fibrous tissue at the mandibular suture or symphysis. At birth, the body of the mandible is relatively large, with alveolar processes similar to those discussed previously in the maxilla, that contain the dental buds for the deciduous teeth as well as those for many of the permanent teeth that are located internal to the deciduous teeth. In the newborn infant, the ramus, which is the more vertical portion of the mandible, is short and broad and at about a 140-145 degree angle to the body. At the top of the ramus are projections called the condyloid and coronoid processes. Cartilage on the posterosuperior aspect of the condyloid process articulates with a

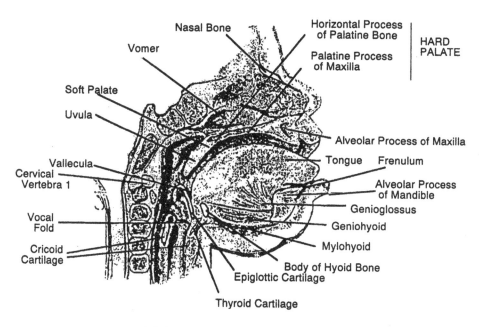

FIGURE 2.13. Adapted from Bosma 1986 (figure 2.14).

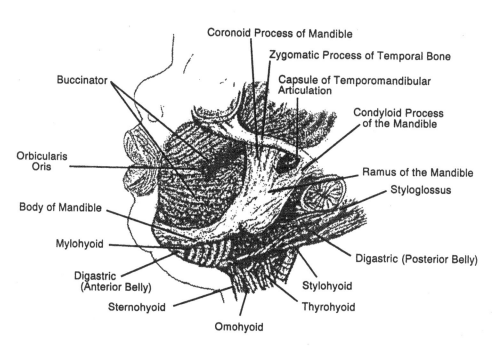

FIGURE 2.14. Adapted from Bosma 1986 (figure 6.19).

slightly indented cavity of the temporal bone to form the temporomandibular joint or articulation. Since there is no true articular eminence at the point where the condyle and skull meet in the infant, the temporomandibular articulation is more mobile in its anterior-posterior and lateral planes. Generally, the normal newborn infant's mandible is in a slightly retracted position relative to the maxilla.

Functionally, the mandible directly and indirectly relates to the skull, cheeks, lips, tongue, maxilla, hyoid bone, epiglottis, pharynx, larynx, thyroid, and shoulder girdle through skeletal, muscular, nerve, and fascial connections. The muscles of the mandible are generally viewed in terms of their roles in its opening or depression (lateral pterygoid, digastric, mylohyoid, and geniohyoid muscles) and its closure or elevation (masseter, medial pterygoid, and temporalis muscles). However, these muscles also should be recognized in regard to their positional stabilization of the mandible as well as their assistance in moving the mandible in up-down, forward-backward, lateral, diagonal, and circular dimensions in conjunction with its mobility at the temporomandibular joint.

The skin, panniculus, fascia, connective tissue, and musculature of the newborn's face, specifically in the area of the cheeks and lips, provide stability for the more mobile structures of the oral mechanism (Bosma 1986). The panniculus, composed of irregularly-sized fat masses that develop throughout the body during the last few months before birth, is particularly thick at the cheeks and adheres directly to the thick, firm layer of skin also found in this area of the face. Within the cheeks, lying between the buccinator and masseter muscles, are the buccal, or sucking, fat pads. They are encapsulated masses of dense fatty tissue different in composition from the panniculus. These buccal pads appear to provide added stability to the area of the cheeks during the infant's suckling and sucking activity. Although the panniculus persists into early childhood, the buccal fat pads appear to exist in some degree throughout adulthood.

The buccal fat pads approximate the buccinator muscle, which is substantial in its mass within the newborn infant's cheeks. The buccinator muscle is continuous with the orbicularis oris muscle of the lips, inferiorly, and the superior pharyngeal constrictor, posteriorly. Anteriorly, it attaches to the alveolar processes of the mandible and maxilla. The buccal cavity or space within the infant's oral cavity is small due to the small vertical distance between the alveolar processes of the mandible and maxilla and the limited lateral mobility of the cheeks, which is created by the buccal fat pads and thick panniculus.

The infant's lips are vertically short in comparison to the anterior aspects of the maxilla and mandible, to which they attach. On the inner surface of each lip is a fold of mucous membrane connecting the lip to the gums. This membrane is called the median frenulum. In the newborn, it extends over most of its vertical length. The labial sulci or spaces between the lips and their corresponding skeletal attachments at the maxilla and mandible are very shallow.

The cheeks and lips meet at the nasolabial folds, which are distinctive in the newborn as they distinguish the less mobile cheeks from the more mobile lips. Muscle fibers of the orbicularis oris insert into the skin at the middle of the upper lip, contributing to the formation of the "Cupid's bow" and the indentation superior to it called the philtrum.

The lips of the newborn are generally positioned in an outward or everted contour that increases during activities such as breastfeeding, bottledrinking, and crying. The lower lip appears more mobile than the upper lip, passively as well as during feeding and crying activities.

The muscle of the lips is the sphincter-like orbicularis oris, which generally functions in lip protrusion and rounding as well as lip closure. In the newborn, the orbicularis oris appears to assist in narrowing or constricting the lips positionally around the nipple. Other musculature that will influence lip activity in the future include the depressor anguli oris (triangularis), depressor labii inferioris (quadratus labii inferioris), and mentalis that assist in lower lip depression; the levator anguli oris (canine), quadratus labii superioris, and zygomatic major that assist in upper lip elevation; the buccinator, risorius, and platysma that assist in lip spreading; the incisivis labii superior that draws the mouth corners upward and medially; and the incisivis labii inferior that draws the mouth corners downward and medially. As these muscles become more active, they not only directly effect movements of the cheeks and lips, but also provide active stability essential for the further development of jaw and tongue movements.

The tongue of the newborn infant fills the oral cavity. At rest, it approximates the lower lip, anteriorly; the alveolar ridge of the mandible and the inner wall of the cheeks, laterally; the hard palate, superiorly; and the soft palate and epiglottis, posteriorly.

The infant's tongue is relatively short and broad in size. The body of the tongue is composed of intrinsic musculature and fascia, an aponeurosis, and a mucosal covering. The mucosa on the superior surface of the oral portion of the tongue body (dorsum of the tongue) has many types of papillae containing the taste buds.

Changing the shape or contour of the tongue is the primary role of the four intrinsic tongue muscles. The superior longitudinal muscles shorten the tongue and curl its tip and lateral margins upward, giving a concave appearance to the tongue's dorsum.

The inferior longitudinal muscles curl the tip downward and, when working in conjunction with the superior longitudinal muscles, can retract, shorten, and widen the tongue. The transverse muscles narrow and elongate the tongue. The vertical muscles flatten the tongue and when working in conjunction with the transverse muscles, can increase the length of the tongue.

Although the muscles, fascia, aponeurosis, and mucosa of the tongue body provide it with a foundation of internal stability, the tongue depends on its extrinsic musculature to provide an essential framework of physical support and stabilization as well as to assist in movement. The shortness in length and arrangement of the extrinsic tongue musculature in the infant provides an important point of stability from which the tongue can be positioned and moved.

Through its extrinsic muscles (figure 2.15), the tongue is directly related to the styloid process of the temporal bone (styloglossus), hyoid bone (hyoglossus), man-dible (genioglossus), and soft palate (palatoglossus), creating a system of support and alignment from which the oral mechanism can function. The styloglossus draws the tongue backward and upward, while the genioglossus depresses the tongue, forming a trough-like configuration. Raising of the back of the tongue or lowering of the soft palate occurs dependent on which structure is more firmly fixed in position through the contraction of the palatoglossus. Retraction and depression of the tongue body or elevation of the hyoid bone results from the actions of the hyoglossus dependent on whether the hyoid bone or tongue is more securely positioned. Although the tongue is most often discussed in terms of its role as part of the oral mechanism, its posterior portion, which lies within the pharynx, reflects its importance to the functions of both the oral and pharyngeal areas.

The pharyngeal mechanism. The pharyngeal cavity or pharynx (figure 2.16) is a musculomembranous tube that extends downward from the sphenoid bone at the base of the skull to the laryngeal and esophageal openings. Generally, the pharynx is described in terms of its three sections: the nasopharynx, oropharynx, and laryngopharynx. The nasopharynx is the area upward from the soft palate to the base of the skull including the opening to the nasal cavity. The oropharynx extends from the soft palate downward to the hyoid bone and is continuous with the oral cavity. The laryngopharynx is the area from the hyoid bone down to the openings of the larynx and esophagus. Since the newborn infant's pharynx is short (approximately one-third the length of the adult pharynx), with approximation of many of its positionally-elevated structures, and is curved in its overall shape, it is more difficult to differentiate among its sections when compared to the more elongated and angled pharyngeal cavities of the child and the adult.

In terms of the normal developmental process regarding functional activities, our discussion of the structures and musculature of the pharyngeal cavity focuses on those most significantly associated with feeding, swallowing, and respiration and includes additional information on the larynx and esophagus pertinent to these functions. More specific information on the larynx and its relationship to sound production is described in Chapter 8.

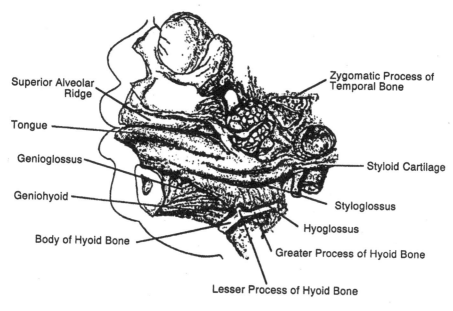

FIGURE 2.15. Adapted from Bosma 1986 (figure 6.20).

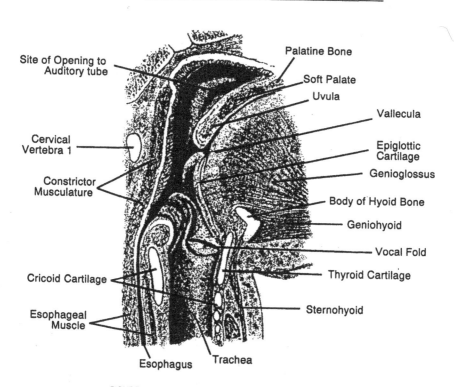

FIGURE 2.16. Adapted from Bosma 1986 (figure 2.35).

The constrictor muscles that make up the lateral and posterior walls of the pharynx anteriorly attach to the skeleton of the face, structures of the oral cavity, the larynx, and the hyoid and are continuous with other musculature and fascia of the face and pharyngeal area. The three constrictor muscles are referred to as the superior, middle, and inferior pharyngeal constrictors. Each muscle courses from its anterior attachment posteriorly in the lateral and posterior walls, meeting its opposite muscle at the median raphe. In the newborn infant these muscles can be differentiated from each other in the lateral wall of the pharynx but not in the posterior wall. It is not until the pharyngeal cavity elongates and its structures descend that these constrictor muscles can be distinguished in the posterior wall of the pharynx. The constrictor muscles make the walls of the pharynx mobile and, upon contraction, constrict the pharyngeal cavity, creating the peristaltic movement needed to propel food down to the esophagus.

The inferior pharyngeal constrictor is often referred to in terms of its two muscular segments: the thyropharyngeus and the cricopharyngeus. The cricopharyngeus is of particular importance in regard to its continuous relationship with the circular muscle at the entrance to the esophagus (the upper esophageal sphincter, UES, p-e segment), contributing to its constriction of the opening. This is essential for preventing air from entering the esophagus and gastric contents from refluxing into the pharynx.

The wall of the pharyngeal cavity also has internal longitudinal muscles, including the salpingopharyngeus, palatopharyngeus, palatolaryngeus, and stylopharyngeus. Only the stylopharyngeus has an attachment outside the pharynx on the styloid process of the temporal bone. After the pharyngeal mechanism has begun to elongate in later infancy, the salpingopharyngeus and palatopharyngeus motorically act in sequence with contraction of the levator veli palatini as it lifts the soft palate up and back toward the posterior pharyngeal wall for velopharyngeal closure. Significant to crying and swallowing, these longitudinal muscles appear to have a primary role in shortening the vertical dimension of the pharynx below the level of the soft palate while assisting in its constriction. It has been inferred that the salpingopharyngeus and stylopharyngeus muscles may assist in displacing the pharyngeal wall, creating the significant enlargement of the infant's pharynx that occurs with effortful inspirations during crying (Bosma 1986).

The pharynx and upper airway essentially are suspended from the base of the skull. However, through muscles that attach to the hyoid bone and the larynx, a system of support exists that allows the pharynx to play a central role in feeding, swallowing, sound production, airway maintenance, and the development of head and neck control (Kramer 1985).

The muscles that provide this support framework, especially once the infant begins to grow and the pharynx begins to elongate, are the suprahyoid and infrahyoid muscles (see figures 2.14 and 2.15, pages 23 and 27). The suprahyoid muscles, which assist in elevating the hyoid bone and larynx, include the digastric, mylohyoid, and geniohyoid, which also act as depressors of the mandible; the hyoglossus and genioglossus, which act as part of the extrinsic tongue musculature; and the stylohyoid, which connects the hyoid to the base of the skull. The infrahyoid muscles, which assist in depressing the hyoid bone and larynx, are the sternohyoid, omohyoid, sternothyroid, and thyrohyoid. They attach the hyoid bone to the sternum, clavicles, scapulae, ribs, and thyroid, creating an important point of stability for the pharyngeal area from below. When elements of the suprahyoids and infrahyoids work in cooperation, the hyoid bone can be fixed in position. As the infant's development progresses, these muscles also play a role in achieving active neutral head flexion with neck elongation.

Within the nasopharynx, at the level of the floor of the nasal cavity and near the junction of the hard and soft palates, are the openings into the auditory, or eustachian, tubes. In the newborn, the eustachian tubes are almost horizontal in placement and their openings into the nasopharynx are relatively small (Crelin 1973). The pharyngeal openings of the tubes protrude into the nasopharynx, remaining closed except when opened by muscle contraction such as occurs during swallowing. The position of the opening of the eustachian tubes in the nasopharynx and their horizontal orientation increase the infant's risk for middle ear infections.

Although the tongue is generally considered an oral structure, its influences on the pharynx are significant. The mass of the tongue body, the attachments of its extrinsic musculature, and its movements during functional activities impact on the alignment, contour, and movements of the anterior aspects of the oropharynx and laryngopharynx. In the newborn infant, the internal stabilization provided by the close approximation of the tongue to the hard palate, soft palate, and epiglottis also influences the position and alignment of the larynx. The extrinsic tongue musculature of the infant is an essential element in the maintenance of the upper airway. After the posterior third of the infant's tongue begins to gradually descend to its future place as part of the anterior pharyngeal wall, changes in the alignment, contour, and movements of the tongue and other pharyngeal and laryngeal structures occur.

The structures of the oropharynx and laryngopharynx are high in position and vertically compact within the cervical area. The epiglottis is a flexible, thin fibrocartilaginous structure covered by a thick submucosa. Although it is usually short in the newborn, it extends slightly into the oropharynx in the shape of a flattened blade or an upside-down trough. Its distal end approximates the uvula, limiting the size of the infant's oropharynx. The valleculae are the spaces bordered by the epiglottis, tongue, and lateral walls of the pharynx in which liquid accumulates during suckling until the pharyngeal swallow is initiated.

The hyoid bone in the newborn infant is higher in position and more horizontal in orientation than is found in the child and adult. Although primarily composed of cartilage, the central portion of the body of the hyoid may be ossified in the newborn infant. The hyoid bone is in the shape of an arch and is composed of three parts: the body, the greater processes, and the lesser processes.

The hyoid bone has several distinctive roles. It serves as a primary skeletal attachment for fascia and musculature of the pharynx, tongue, and larynx. Through its suprahyoid and infrahyoid musculature attachments, it is directly associated with the mandible, tongue, styloid process, larynx, shoulder girdle, and upper rib cage. Therefore, it not only contributes to movements of the oral, pharyngeal, and laryngeal areas, but also to their alignment with the head, neck, shoulder girdle, and rib cage. The hyoid moves with the tongue and larynx for swallowing, actively participates in respiration, and assists in maintaining the pharyngeal airway.

The thyroid cartilage of the infant's larynx is within and slightly inferior to the arch of the hyoid bone, joined at its superior cornua to the posterior end of the greater processes of the hyoid by a flexible ligament. The inferior cornua of the thyroid cartilage articulate with the cricoid cartilage through a broad fibrous attachment. The cricoid cartilage is the foundation of the larynx situated in the area where the pharynx, esophagus, trachea, and arytenoid cartilages meet. The arytenoid cartilages, which the vocal folds attach to posteriorly, articulate with the cricoid cartilage on its posterosuperior margin.

The piriform recesses, or sinuses, are depressions in the posterior laryngopharynx lateral to the cricoid and arytenoid cartilages and medial to the thyroid cartilage in which secretions and residual liquid or food may accumulate. With the larynx elevated and closed with upward compression during the swallow, this material is prevented from entering the laryngeal vestibule, or supraglottic space, in the young infant.

Rib cage and diaphragm. The round contour and more horizontal placement of the ribs and the elevated position of the newborn infant's rib cage are reflected in the cylindrical shape of the chest with anterior-posterior and transverse diameters that are approximately equal in size (Green and Doershuk 1985). The diaphragm, which is the primary muscle of inspiration used by the newborn infant, is positioned higher in the thoracic cavity at rest, allowing for its more efficient use on inspiration.

The skeletal framework of the rib cage consists of the ribs, sternum, and thoracic spine (figure 2.17). Twelve ribs on either side of the spine articulate posteriorly with the thoracic vertebrae. The upper seven ribs, often called the true or vertebro-sternal ribs, attach anteriorly to the sternum through the costal cartilages. The remaining five ribs, or the false ribs, are divided into the first three (vertebro-chondral ribs), which attach anteriorly to the cartilage of the rib above, and the last two (floating or vertebral ribs), which have no anterior attachments. The sternum or breastbone is divided into the manubrium, sternal body, and xiphoid process.

At birth, the ribs and sternum are primarily cartilaginous in composition. This gives them greater flexibility and makes the ribs and sternum less resistant to forces placed upon them by surrounding musculature activity.

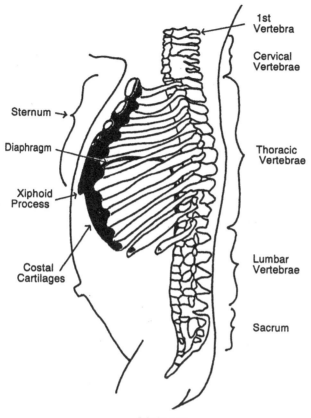

FIGURE 2.17.
Adapted from Crelin 1969 (figure 9).

The diaphragm is a musculotendinous sheet composed of a central tendon surrounded by muscle tissue. It separates the thoracic and abdominal cavities and forms the floor of the thoracic cavity. The diaphragm originates from the posterior aspect of the xiphoid process of the sternum, the inner surfaces of the costal cartilages and adjacent aspects of the last six ribs, and the first and second lumbar vertebrae.

When relaxed, the diaphragm is dome shaped. With contraction of its musculature on inspiration, the central aspects of the diaphragm flatten, the abdominal wall is pushed outward, and the lower ribs are pulled up and move outward, resulting in lower rib expansion or rib flaring. Forceful contraction of the diaphragm may result in retraction or inward movement of the sternum and lower rib cage, which decreases the efficiency of the diaphragm and reduces the tidal volume, or volume of air that can actually be used by the infant.

The diaphragm also has been found to exhibit postinspiratory activity. This assists the newborn infant in slowing or prolonging expiration so that an appropriate volume of air can be maintained in the respiratory tract when at resting position

(Functional Respiratory Capacity). When this occurs, the diaphragm continues to be active for a brief period at the start of expiration as a holding action. This is sufficient to oppose the elastic recoil of expiratory forces and allows the infant to hold peak inspiratory volume for a longer time (Davis and Bureau 1987).

Although the muscles of the rib cage are not used by the newborn infant to expand the thoracic cavity during inspiration, they are discussed in terms of providing stability to the chest wall during diaphragmatic contraction (Davis and Bureau 1987). These muscles, which help resist rib cage distortion, include the external and internal intercostals; the sternocleidomastoids; the pectoralis major and minor; the scaleni anterior, medius, and posterior; the serratus anterior; and the subclavius.

Developmental Characteristics

The oral, pharyngeal, and respiratory mechanisms modify as the infant uses them functionally. Feeding and sound production are two primary activities in which these developmental changes occur. However, other influences also impact on the infant's development in oral-motor and respiratory function.

When in prone with the head turned to the side, sensory input is provided to the face and cheeks by the surface the newborn infant is lying on (figure 2.18). As the newborn lifts and turns the head in prone, the lips and cheeks often make contact with the surface. When held or positioned so that the hand comes in contact with the mouth, the newborn infant sucks or suckles on it. These early sensory-motor experiences also play a significant role in the infant's development of active movements of the oral, pharyngeal, and respiratory mechanisms.

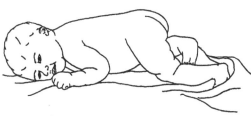

FIGURE 2.18.

The feeding process. The oral and pharyngeal mechanisms of the newborn have been prepared for the feeding process during fetal development. Sucking and swallowing may be elicited in fetal development as early as 17 weeks and 29 weeks, respectively. The coordination of sucking, swallowing, and breathing, which is essential for safe, efficient oral feeding, is present at approximately 34 weeks gestational age. The gag response, inconsistently seen as early as 26-27 weeks gestational age, is not consistently present until at least 32-33 weeks gestation. The ability to cough may be elicited at 26-27 weeks, although it is not consistently functional until approximately 37-38 weeks gestation. Therefore, the full-term newborn infant has the ability to engage in feeding and swallowing activities at birth.

The newborn infant exhibits automatic responses stimulated through tactile input, which are related to the feeding process. The rooting response is characterized by turning the head and movements of the jaw, tongue, and lips toward touch on the cheeks and lips. It is considered a food-seeking movement since it is strongest when the infant is hungry or held in the position generally used for feeding. The automatic phasic bite-release pattern is elicited by touch to the biting surface of the gums, resulting in small vertical up and down jaw movements similar to those used to pump liquid from the nipple. The gag response, important for the protection of the airway, is stimulated by tactile input to the posterior tongue or oral cavity, resulting in head extension, jaw depression, tongue protrusion, and constriction of the pharyngeal area. Of these three automatic responses, only the gag response is modified in its strength and retained throughout adulthood.

Initially, the anatomical framework and physiological state of the newborn infant provides a foundation of internal stability that is directly reflected in breastfeeding and bottledrinking. Orally, the tongue, jaw, cheeks, and lips work together as a unit. The extent of vertical jaw movements is restricted by the jaw's proximity to the high-positioned rib cage; influences of physiological flexion at the head, neck, and shoulder girdle; and stability provided by the sucking fat pads of the cheeks. The tongue remains within the oral mechanism, moves up and down with the jaw, and cups around the nipple. The lips positionally surround the nipple without actively holding onto it. This pattern of oral movements is often referred to as a true sucking pattern, or a total pattern of sucking, differentiating it from active sucking that the infant will develop in the future and that requires coordinated musculature activity of the cheeks, lips, tongue, and jaw (figure 2.19).

As the newborn infant begins to develop antigravity head extension, movements of the oral mechanism begin to modify. The jaw moves up/down and forward/backward in large rhythmical movements to pump the liquid from the bottle or breast. The tongue rhythmically moves with the jaw in a forward/backward direction, stroking the nipple in more of a licking type of movement. The lips continue to be postured forward to surround the nipple but may not be able to keep constant contact with it due to the movements of the jaw and tongue. This new active pattern of oral movement is called suckling (figure 2.20).

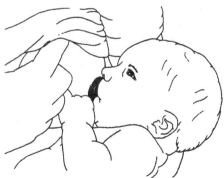

FIGURE 2.19

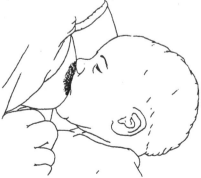

FIGURE 2.20

Since the lips are not actively holding on the nipple, liquid might be lost during breastfeeding and bottledrinking. Less liquid loss is noted when an infant is breastfed because the breast more accurately conforms to the posture of the lips even when larger movements of the jaw are evident.

As the infant's tongue and jaw rhythmically compress the nipple up against the hard palate, negative pressure is created that brings the liquid back in the oral cavity. A swallow is initiated, moving liquid from the valleculae around the epiglottis and down into the esophagus.

Due to the arrangement of the oral and pharyngeal structures and musculature, the newborn infant is an obligatory nose breather. This skeletal and muscular arrangement as well as the movements of the oral, pharyngeal, and laryngeal mechanisms physically protect the opening to the larynx as liquid is swallowed. Therefore, the infant can coordinate breathing with suckling and swallowing activities.

The way that an infant is held during feeding can influence the pattern of oral movements used, especially once head extension is being developed. If the infant's head is positioned downward toward the elevated rib cage, the jaw is restricted in the size of its excursions. Oral movements like those noted in a total pattern of sucking, with greater negative pressure within the oral cavity, are produced. If the infant's head is permitted to extend slightly, jaw and tongue movements are more characteristic of suckling. The infant's opportunity to experience a variety of oral movements will assist in the future development of more controlled, active oral-motor function.

Significant components of respiratory function. The respiratory pattern of the newborn infant is a belly breathing pattern (diaphragmatic or abdominal breathing). When at rest or during quiet breathing, expansion of the belly is evident on inspiration with no apparent rib cage movement (figure 2.21). Some infants exhibit slight lower rib expansion as the diaphragm contracts and pulls the lower ribs upward and outward.

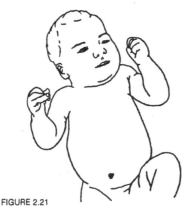

FIGURE 2.21

Effortful movement, crying, and other stressful activities affect the infant's belly breathing pattern. Although belly expansion occurs, the forceful contraction of the diaphragm that accompanies more stressful inspiration pulls on the flexible rib cage. This often produces a collapse or inward movement of the anterior rib cage with sternal retraction especially observable at the xiphoid process. The rectus abdominus muscle may bulge outward when extreme effort is involved (figure 2.22). Lower rib expansion or rib flaring also occurs.

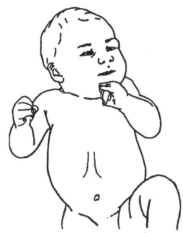

FIGURE 2.22

Immediately after birth, infants begin sustained, rhythmical breathing. This does not mean that the rhythmicity of an infant's breathing is always the same. Asynchrony in the breathing rhythm occurs when the newborn infant is engaged in effortful activity and crying. Periodic breathing, which is characterized by brief apneic periods or respiratory pauses of 3 seconds or greater that are interrupted by respirations of 20 seconds or less in duration, can be seen in the normal, healthy infant especially during the first few weeks of life (Richmond and Galgoczy 1979). The normal newborn infant's respiratory rate is described as variable at 30-60 breaths per minute with an average rate of 30-40 breaths per minute.

The infant is able to create phonation or generate voiced sound, which is produced when the true vocal folds of the larynx adduct just enough to vibrate as air pressure pushes against them. Phonation such as crying or other vowel-like sounds are produced by the infant primarily on exhalation. Crying is generally characterized by a rising pitch and a nasal quality.

Other sounds are produced by the infant with general body movements and during feeding as the oral mechanism moves, interrupting or modifying the airflow. Voiceless consonant-like sounds including clicks and friction noises of short duration and low intensity are often heard.

A direct relationship exists between the production of sound and movement of the body by the infant (figure 2.23). As the infant moves, the internal foundation needed to generate laryngeal activity in coordination with respiratory air flow is stimulated. This pairing of sound production with body movement continues until the infant is at least eight to nine months of age.

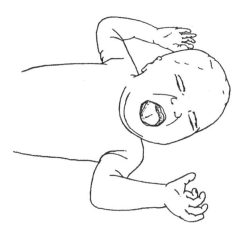

FIGURE 2.23

See Chapter 8 for further information on speech production development.

Summary Chart–Newborn

Postural Control	Gross Motor	Reach	Fine Motor	Vision	Oral-Motor/Feeding	Respiration-Phonation
Physiological flexion—provides stability for posture and random movements	Movements limited by available range of motion	Random arm movements within a 90-degree plane	Strong grasp reflex	Visual regard for environment	Strong gag response, rooting response, and automatic phasic bite-release pattern	*Respiration* Obligatory nose breather
Neck righting	Random movements	Positional hand-to-hand contact and reflexive hand-to-mouth contact in sidelying	Hands open as arms abduct	Random, disorganized eye movements	*Feeding* On bottle/breast, starts with true sucking pattern using total pattern of oral movements	Belly breathing at rest and during quiet breathing
Labyrinthine righting beginning in prone and supine	• rhythmical alternating movements of limbs			Monocular vision	Begins suckling movements of oral area after antigravity head extension starts developing	Belly breathing with anterior rib cage collapse/sternal retraction during stressful/effortful activities and crying
Primary standing reaction	• total body movements into extension or flexion				Mixture of suckling/sucking on bottle/breast dependent on head position when held	Sustained, rhythmical breathing generally; asynchronous rhythm with effortful activity/crying
	• primitive reactions elicited by a specific stimulus				*Oral-Motor* Suckles/sucks when hand/object comes in contact with mouth	*Phonation/Sounds* Direct relationship between phonation/sound production and body movement
	• distal isolated movements				Minimal drooling in supine or when reclined; increased drooling in other positions	Produces cry or vowel-like sounds primarily on exhalation; nasal in quality
	Lifts and turns head part way in prone					Produces clicks/friction noises of short duration and low intensity
	Automatic stepping					

Some infants develop activities earlier or later than this chart indicates. Therefore, it should not be regarded as a rigid timetable of events.

■ References

Bly, L. 1983. *The components of normal movement during the first year of life and abnormal motor development.* Chicago: Neuro-Developmental Treatment Association.

Bosma, J. F. 1986. *Anatomy of the infant head.* Baltimore: The Johns Hopkins University Press.

Caplan, F. 1971. *The first twelve months of life.* New York: Grosset and Dunlap.

Crelin, E. S. 1969. *Anatomy of the newborn: An atlas.* Philadelphia: Lea & Febiger.

———. 1973. *Functional anatomy of the newborn.* New Haven, CT: Yale University Press.

Davis, G. M., and M. A. Bureau. 1987. Pulmonary and chest wall mechanics in the control of respiration in the newborn. In *Clinics in perinatology*, Vol. 14, edited by L. Stern, 551-79. Philadelphia: W. B. Saunders.

Erhardt, R. P. 1982. *Developmental hand dysfunction: Theory, assessment, and treatment.* Tucson, AZ: Therapy Skill Builders.

———. 1990. *Developmental visual dysfunction models for assessment and management.* Tucson, AZ: Therapy Skill Builders.

Green, C. C., and C. F. Doershuk. 1985. Development of the respiratory system. In *Pediatric respiratory therapy*, edited by M. D. Lough, C. F. Doershuk, and R. C. Stern, 1-24. Chicago: Year Book Medical Publishers, Inc.

Jan, J. E., R. D. Freeman, and E. P. Scott. 1987. *Visual impairment in children and adolescents.* New York: Grune and Stratton.

Kamm, K., E. Thelen, and J. Jensen. 1990. A dynamical systems approach to motor development. *Physical Therapy* 70:763-75.

Kramer, S. S. 1985. Special swallowing problems in children. *Gastrointestinal Radiology* 10:241-50.

Maurer, D., and C. Maurer. 1988. *The world of the newborn.* New York: Basic Books, Inc.

Myklebust, B. 1990. A review of myotatic reflexes and the development of motor control and gait in infants and children: A special communication. *Physical Therapy* 70:188-203.

Netter, F. H. 1979. Respiratory system. In *CIBA collection of medical illustrations*, Vol. 7, edited by M. Divertie and A. Brass, 3-43. Summit, NJ: CIBA Pharmaceutical.

Norkin, C., and P. Levangie. 1983. *Joint structure and function*. Philadelphia: F. A. Davis.

Perkins, W. H., and R. D. Kent. 1986. *Functional anatomy of speech, language, and hearing: A primer*. Waltham, MA: College-Hill Press/Little, Brown & Co.

Richmond, B., and M. Galgoczy. 1979. Development of the cardiorespiratory system. In *Newborn respiratory care*, edited by M. D. Lough, T. J. Williams, and J. E. Rawson, 1-48. Chicago: Year Book Medical Publishers, Inc.

Weggemenn, T., J. K. Brown, G. E. Fulford, and R. A. Minns. 1987. A study of normal baby movements. *Child: Care, Health and Development* 13:41-58.

Chapter 3

1-2 Months

■ Postural Control

Physiological flexion diminishes so that during the second month the infant may seem relatively hypotonic as active postural control is only beginning. When pulled to sitting, there may be a greater head lag than in the newborn period when flexor tone and immobility kept the head close to the shoulders (figure 3.1); however, by the end of the second month, asymmetrical flexion may be seen. Head righting continuously develops from birth and is seen as the infant lifts the head higher in prone. Also, when tipped forward or backward, the baby attempts to get the head upright, but is unable to maintain it as flexor and extensor control are not yet working together. Until this occurs, the head bobs and lateral control cannot develop.

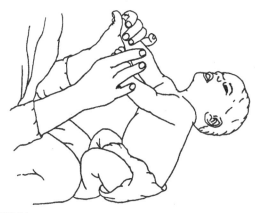

FIGURE 3.1

During the second month, the infant can be held upright to an adult's shoulder, the body conforming to the shoulder and the head turning to rest on it for support. The infant also lifts the head off the adult's shoulder and holds it upright momentarily (figure 3.2); this ability increases throughout the second month. Although the infant requires support, spinal extensors provide some trunk stability, which is required for head control. Babies with lower postural tone may take longer to develop upright control of the head as they do not have sufficient stability of the trunk and shoulder girdle.

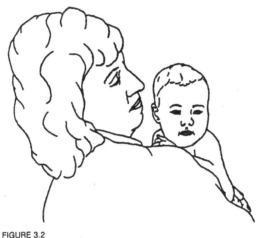

FIGURE 3.2

■ Gross Motor Development

Anatomical/Structural Characteristics

The most significant changes in spinal mobility are increased extension of the thoracic and upper lumbar areas and increased cervical and upper thoracic rotation. Studies reveal extremely variable ranges of lower extremity motion in infants, partially due to a lack of standardization of testing methods. Hip extension and abduction increases, but changes in rotation have not been consistently documented. Although the combined functional range of flexion/abduction/external rotation increases, it is not clear whether a larger range of abduction allows this pattern or if other changes in mobility also occur, possibly stretching of the joint capsule by the infant's random movements. This appears to occur at the knee joint as extension increases with the hip both flexed and extended, indicating lengthening of the hamstrings and changes in the joint capsule (Reade et al. 1984).

Posture and Movement

Random movements continue from the newborn period with less reflexive movements, greater excursion, and increased coordination of rhythmical patterns. Movements are less jerky with improved spatial and temporal synchrony of joint motions. For example, the hip and knee flex and extend together, resulting in a smoother kicking pattern in a shorter period of time. The head and extremities appear more free as they begin to be disassociated from the trunk.

Supine posture is generally more extended and still asymmetrical (figure 3.3). The infant easily turns the head from side to side through a greater excursion, but is unable to hold it in midline. Asymmetrical extension is used to rotate the head away from midline and asymmetrical flexion is used to rotate it toward midline. The asymmetrical tonic neck reflex (ATNR) can be observed and serves as a pattern of postural control. The shoulder retraction and flexion of the skull-side arm gives stability for increased head turning. As rotation increases, a weight shift occurs in the trunk, providing asymmetrical tactile and proprioceptive input, which are preliminary to later voluntary rolling. Some infants attempt to lift the head in supine, recruiting a total flexion pattern (neck flexors, pectorals, and rectus abdominus); however, they can lift it only slightly as they cannot tuck the chin or maintain a sufficient contraction of the prevertebral neck muscles.

The infant lies with arms and legs more extended. The newborn baby was able to kick into extension but the feet rarely touched the surface due to hip and knee flexion. However, the two-month-old can rest with the lateral border of the feet on the surface (increased lumbar extension and hip extension/abduction/external rotation).

In prone, the infant works extremely hard at lifting and turning the head (figure 3.4). Initially the baby uses asymmetrical extension to one side, then may turn the head to the other side but is unable to hold or lift in midline.

By the end of the second month, the infant can symmetrically lift the head about 45 degrees. Increased spinal and hip mobility allow the baby's center of gravity to be less on the head and more on the shoulders and upper chest, making head lifting easier. The upper and lower extremities are often actively moving as if the infant needs

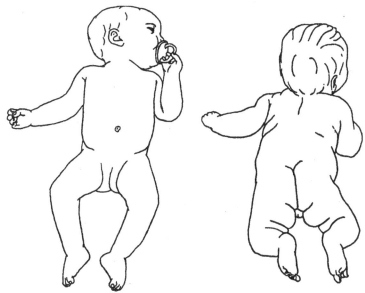

FIGURE 3.3

FIGURE 3.4

momentum to help activate the head and spine. The spinal extensors are very active from the cervical through the lumbar area, although they provide stability more than movement excursion. As active hip flexion/abduction/external rotation mechanically tilts the pelvis anteriorly, the range of lumbar extension is increased.

Placed in sitting position, the one- to two-month-old baby attempts to lift the head, but does not have the stability of prone. The pelvis is perpendicular to the supporting surface and the spine is flexed (figure 3.5). If supported at the trunk, the infant may extend the head and spine but is unable to control it, resulting in a bobbing movement. The infant fatigues easily and falls forward into flexion.

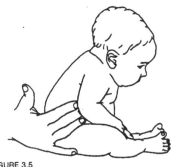

FIGURE 3.5

The infant can be active in a semi-reclined infant seat with less lateral support than required at birth. The posterior trunk is the base of support working off the back surface of the seat. The infant can swipe with the arms, kick the legs, and turn the head at the same time or separately. The infant may begin to hold the head to visually contact an object while moving arms and legs. Extremity movements increase with excitement and vocalization.

Primary standing and automatic stepping diminish and usually cannot be elicited after the first month. The lower extremities appear disorganized and the infant takes little or no weight on the feet or may briefly extend, then collapse.

■ Fine Motor Development

Upper Extremity Development

In prone, the one-month-old baby can asymmetrically lift the head to shoulder level. Medial scapular activity is beginning to develop. There continues to be marked shoulder elevation; however, the small rotator cuff muscles are now strong enough to prevent the complete collapse of shoulders during head lifting that occurred at birth (figure 3.6). Due to greater spinal and hip mobility, the upper body supports less weight than it did at birth. The weight the shoulders do support is distributed between the shoulders and the heels of the fisted hands because the elbows are positioned well behind the shoulders. At rest, the infant's arms begin to abduct and externally rotate, with the hands generally fisted (figure 3.7).

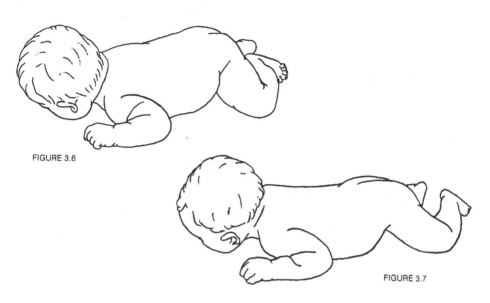

FIGURE 3.6

FIGURE 3.7

The two-month-old baby asymmetrically lifts the head slightly above shoulder level, shifting more weight to the trunk and legs. While lifting the head, the infant pushes down with one arm slightly more than the other, thus lifting one shoulder further off the supporting surface (figure 3.8). The forearms now accept partial body weight because the elbows are further forward or in closer proximity to the shoulders. The ulnar borders of the hands also bear weight because the upper arms are in less internal rotation. The neck and shoulders are not yet strong enough to hold this position for more than a few seconds. The two-month-old baby may not want to stay in prone for long periods of waking time, since it is hard work to move the body and view the world in this position.

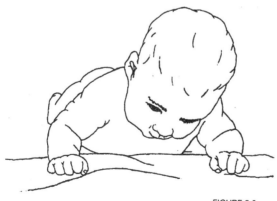

FIGURE 3.8

In supine, the one- to two-month-old randomly moves the arms in wide ranges of shoulder abduction and adduction, but moves them in only a small range of shoulder flexion. This range of motion is possible because the head, scapula, and spine are maintained against the supporting surface. Gravity and the infant's own movements help expand the chest, lengthening the pectoralis major and minor (figure 3.9). Progressively greater shoulder girdle depression is seen as the infant matures. The asymmetry (ATNR) seen at this age is partially initiated with symmetrical activation of scapular adduction (figure 3.10).

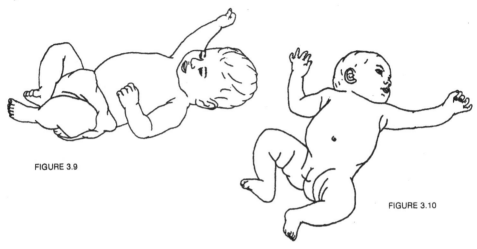

FIGURE 3.9

FIGURE 3.10

One-month-old infants exhibit random arm movements in response to the generalized extension experience throughout the whole body. They do not randomly move their arms in specific response to a visual stimulus. However, at two months of age, they do elicit specific physical responses to visual stimulation. When they are in the process of random motion and a visual stimulus is presented, the body becomes still. On the other hand, when the body is still and a visual stimulus is presented, their arms move randomly and their hands open and close reflexively. Consequently, when a visual stimulus is presented, the two-month-old responds with a shift in physical state.

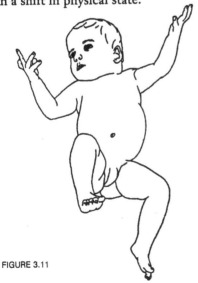

The arm movements of the two-month-old mimic a windmill-type motion. For example, as one arm moves down, the other moves up (figure 3.11). This motion reflects development of the shoulder girdle. The infant's shoulders function as a single unit because the scapulae are not yet dynamically stable on the rib cage. In months to come, the development of more mature prone propping skills will generate dynamic stability in the shoulders and, therefore, will alter the nature of arm movements during reach.

FIGURE 3.11

Hand Development

At this stage of development, the infant continues to exhibit a grasp reflex. The one-month-old infant is unaware that an object is in the hand. After the object is placed, the infant may immediately release it without voluntary control. It is now easier for an adult to pry objects out of the baby's hand than it was at birth.

Conversely, when an object is placed in the hand of the two-month-old, the baby does have some awareness of it and retains the object briefly (figure 3.12). Like the one-month-old infant, the two-month-old baby releases it without voluntary control. One- to two-month-old infants reflexively scratch and clutch tactile input such as a crib blanket or the mother's breast. As they do this, the whole arm tends to pull into flexion.

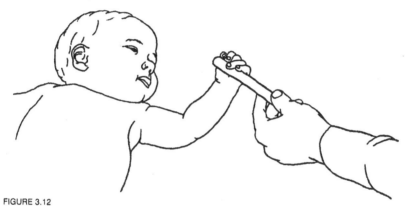

FIGURE 3.12

Visual Development

The one-month-old infant can fixate or steady the gaze and hold it briefly on an object. The infant is most successful with an agitated target, since immobile objects still tend to disappear into background patterns. Visual responses are more consistent when a large object is presented in line with the infant's vision at a 10- to 20-inch distance. The infant exhibits slow, jerky visual tracking from periphery to midline and back to the side using alternating monocular fixation and using one eye or the other (Erhardt 1990). The more interesting the pattern, the longer the duration of gaze. The human face with animated, changing expressions is one of the best stimuli for the one-month-old infant. The baby may also briefly fixate on the hand during random motion.

The two-month-old infant begins inconsistently using binocular fixation, which is the ability to use both eyes simultaneously to focus on a target and fuse the two images into a single perception (Erhardt 1990). Since the baby cannot grade this action, the eyes tend to overconverge or cross slightly. The baby is now aware of movement in the periphery and turns the head and eyes in the direction of the target. The infant can now track slightly past midline using head rotation; however, there is difficulty regulating the speed of eye movements with the speed of the moving target. As the posture moves into an ATNR, the infant maintains a strong visual fixation on one hand, actively using one eye only. The two-month-old infant begins to visually track in a vertical direction as well.

■ Oral-Motor and Respiratory Development

Anatomical/Structural Characteristics

Oral and pharyngeal mechanisms. The size, contour, and alignment of the structures of the oral and pharyngeal mechanisms in the one- to two-month-old infant are essentially the same as discussed for the newborn. Changes in these structures begin to occur at three to five months of age.

Rib cage and diaphragm. The rib cage of the one- to two-month-old infant is comparable to that of the newborn baby. However, greater mobility between the ribs and spine becomes more evident as the infant begins to develop extension of the thoracic spine at two months of age.

Although primary discussion of the respiratory mechanism focuses on the rib cage, diaphragm, and respiratory musculature, some comments regarding the lungs and their composition are appropriate at this time. Green and Doershuk (1985) discuss the lungs in terms of respiratory and nonrespiratory structural components. The nonrespiratory structures, or conducting airways, of the lungs include the trachea, right and left main-stem bronchi, segmental and subsegmental bronchi, smaller bronchi and bronchioles, and terminal bronchioles. The respiratory structures of the lungs grow from the terminal bronchioles and consist of the respiratory bronchioles, alveolar ducts, alveolar sacs, and alveoli. Each lobe of the lung has a "characteristic pattern of asymmetric dichotomous branching airways" (Green and Doershuk 1985) that vary in number and length when comparison is made among the lobes of each lung.

The development of the lungs in terms of their respiratory and nonrespiratory portions and the structures that compose these portions, including the epithelium, mucous glands, goblet cells, cartilage, smooth muscle tissue, and connective tissue, is highly complex. Lung development begins at approximately 24 days in the fetus with the appearance of the primitive lung bud. It continues through the appearance of primitive alveolar structures at 26 weeks gestation and progresses with further development of the respiratory portions of the lungs after birth. Major changes in the size and number of respiratory bronchioles and alveolar structures have been noted as early as the first two months of life, reflecting a significant relationship between the use and development of the respiratory mechanism as a whole and the growth and development of the lungs themselves.

Developmental Characteristics

With the loss of physiological flexion, more active lifting of the head, and greater asymmetry especially in supine and prone, the one- to two-month-old infant exhibits greater vertical excursions of the jaw with forward and backward movements of the tongue. As the infant lifts the head and props the body up in prone or moves in supine using asymmetry, the jaw and tongue often show some pull to the side, because the musculature of the jaw and tongue are directly associated with the head, neck, and shoulder girdle (figure 3.13). The infant experiences new movements of the oral mechanism while beginning to actively move the body in supine and prone. Drooling is more evident as the jaw and tongue move in wider excursions without active use of the cheeks and lips.

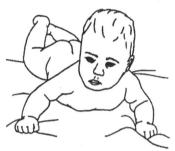

FIGURE 3.13

Like the newborn, the one- to two-month-old infant suckles or sucks when the hand comes in contact with the mouth. These non-nutritive sucking activities provide greater experiences for suckling-swallowing-breathing coordination and oral sensory stimulation. In addition, these rhythmical, non-nutritive sucking activities appear to help the infant organize the body to become calm and quiet.

The feeding process. The jaw and tongue movements used by the one- to two-month-old infant during breastfeeding and bottlefeeding are essentially the same as those used by the newborn infant (figure 3.14). The large, rhythmical, up/down and forward/backward movements of the jaw and rhythmical forward/backward

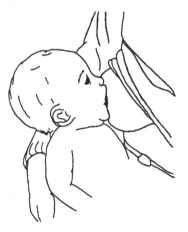

FIGURE 3.14

movements of the tongue characteristic of suckling are predominant as the infant extends and turns the head and extends the neck during feeding (figure 3.15). With increased movement during feeding, the infant may lose coordination of the suckling-swallowing-breathing process, resulting in occasional coughing or choking.

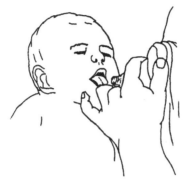

FIGURE 3.15

Significant components of respiratory function. The one- to two-month-old infant continues to use a belly-breathing pattern (figure 3.16). The rib cage is still round in contour and high in position within the trunk. Rib flaring or lower rib expansion is still evident on inhalation as the diaphragm pulls the lower ribs up and out as it contracts, pushing against the abdominal wall.

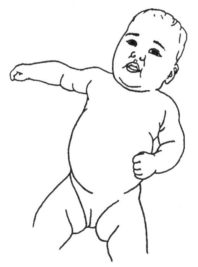

FIGURE 3.16

As the two-month-old moves more actively in prone and supine, changes in rib cage contour may occur in conjunction with belly expansion on inhalation. When the infant moves the arms with a windmill-type motion in supine, the rib cage attached to the arm moving upward elevates with the arm and appears to flatten anteriorly in the area of the pectoralis major (figure 3.17). When kicking the legs in supine, the infant's anterior rib cage (sternum and ribs) may flatten or retract as it is pulled downward and posteriorly with the pull of the rectus abdominus (figure 3.18). With extension of the thoracic spine and greater lifting of the head in prone, rib-to-spine mobility increases and the posterior rib cage contour may appear less rounded (figure 3.19). These changes in rib cage contour with active movement do not prevent the belly expansion that is characteristic of belly breathing, but may affect the rhythm of the infant's breathing making it more asynchronous. Voiced, nasal sounds are often produced on exhalation in direct relationship to the infant's body movements.

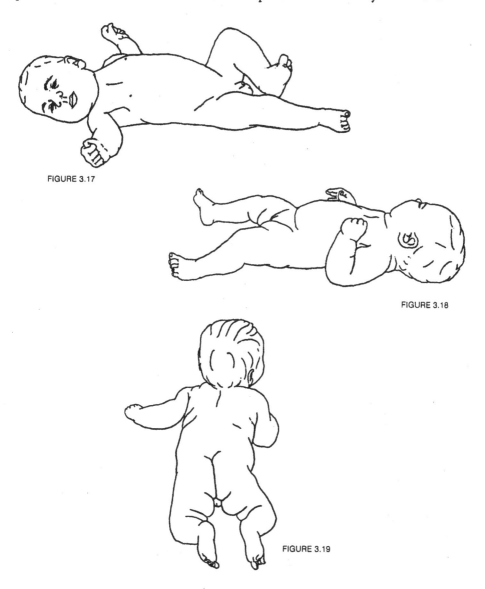

FIGURE 3.17

FIGURE 3.18

FIGURE 3.19

Summary Chart—1-2 Months

Postural Control	Gross Motor	Reach	Fine Motor	Vision	Oral-Motor/Feeding	Respiration-Phonation
Relatively hypotonic as physiological flexion diminishes	Increased range of motion • thoracic and upper lumbar extension • cervical and upper thoracic rotation • hip extension, abduction and flexion/abduction/external rotation • knee extension	Random motion in wider ranges in a horizontal abduction and adduction pattern	Grasp reflex	Monocular fixation	*Respiration* Strong gag response, rooting response, and automatic phasic bite-release pattern	*Respiration* Belly breathing at rest and during quiet breathing; sustained, rhythmical breathing
Head lags in pulled to sit; begins asymmetrical flexion by end of second month	Lifts head in prone 45 degrees by end of second month		Briefly retains object placed in the hand	Tracks from periphery to midline	*Feeding* Suckling movements predominant on bottle/breast; uses some sucking activity	With crying and more active movements in prone and supine, belly breathing with greater lower rib flaring and anterior rib cage flattening/retraction occurs; breathing rhythm may be more asynchronous
Head righting (labrynthine and optical) when tipped forward and backward in space	Rotates head through greater range; in supine, uses asymmetrical posturing to provide stability; lateral weight shift to same side occurs in trunk	Asymmetrical swiping at 2 1/2 months	Reflexively scratches and clutches at blanket	Visually fixates on hand with ATNR	Liquid loss occurs especially with suckling	
	Holds head erect briefly in supported sitting, not steady but bobs				May lose coordination of suckling-swallowing-breathing process with increased head and body movements	*Phonation/Sounds* Cries with greater variations in speed, loudness, duration, pitch, and tension; begins differentiating cry in connection with physiological states
Holds head upright momentarily when trunk is supported	Begins more purposeful movements of arms and legs; uses trunk against the surface for stability			*Some infants develop activities earlier or later than this chart indicates. Therefore, it should not be regarded as a rigid timetable of events.*	*Oral-Motor* Suckles/sucks when hand/object comes in contact with mouth	Produces voiced, nasal vowel sounds in connection with body movement; begins cooing
	Lower extremities disorganized with little or no weight bearing when placed on feet; automatic stepping not elicited				Oral asymmetry evident with asymmetrical extension in supine and prone	
					Drooling increases as jaw and tongue move in wider excursions	

■ References

Erhardt, R. P. 1990. *Developmental visual dysfunction models for assessment and management.* Tucson, AZ: Therapy Skill Builders.

Green, C. C., and C. F. Doershuk. 1985. Development of the respiratory system. In *Pediatric respiratory therapy*, edited by M. D. Lough, C. F. Doershuk, and R. C. Stern, 1-27. Chicago: Year Book Medical Publishers, Inc.

Reade, E., L. Hom, A. Hallum, and R. Lopopolo. 1984. Changes in popliteal angle measurement in infants up to one year of age. *Developmental Medicine and Child Neurology* 26:774-80.

Chapter 4

3-5 Months

■ Postural Control

Head righting is complete by the end of the fifth month, and functional head control is present in all positions. When held upright at three months, the baby maintains the head in a vertical position and, if tipped forward or back, the baby extends or flexes the head and neck accordingly. In the fourth month, lateral flexion occurs when the baby is tilted to the side. By five months, when pulled to a sitting position, the baby flexes and lifts the head, tucking the chin (figure 4.1).

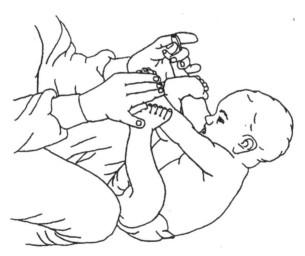

FIGURE 4.1

These head-righting reactions cannot be completely separated from righting reactions of the trunk, which are also active and begin in the third and fourth months. When the infant is tipped in an anterior or posterior direction, extension or flexion of the trunk, respectively, occurs. Forming the basis for control against gravity, similar postural patterns are coordinated functionally with movement as the infant extends to lift the head in prone or flexes to bring hands to the knees in supine. Lateral righting of the trunk can be elicited in the fifth month, but it is not yet an established pattern that can be consistently used in functional movement (figure 4.2).

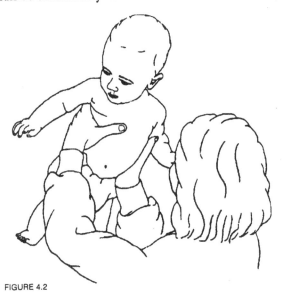

FIGURE 4.2

The four-month-old baby demonstrates the beginning of another type of righting reaction, the Landau. When suspended in a face-down horizontal position, the baby extends the head, neck, and spine accompanied by scapular adduction. In prone the baby uses a similar pattern to play with movement against gravity, lifting the arms and legs off the surface (figure 4.3). Repetition of this activity improves strength, endurance, and coordination for the development of proximal stability, which is the basis for later motor skills. By five to six months, this reaction matures when hip extension is complete and the elbows and knees also have the ability to extend.

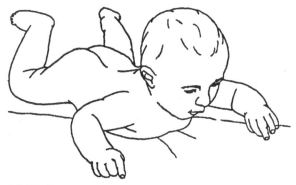

FIGURE 4.3

The infant now begins to establish postural synergies, or a state of readiness in preparation for volitional movement. From three to five months, symmetrical postural activity of proximal musculature provides stability for functional movements to develop in prone and supine. Activity of the erector spinae can be sustained posturally through the sacral area, allowing greater activity in prone, such as head lifting, forearm support, and extended arm support. Simultaneous activity of the prevertebral neck muscles and the spinal extensors, especially in the thoracic area, elongates and stabilizes the spine for independent movements of the head to occur. Together with the pectorals and the abdominals (primarily rectus abdominus), the spinal musculature provides stability for anti-gravity movements of the extremities in supine. Gluteus maximus, medius, and minumus provide hip stability in prone, allowing the center of gravity to shift caudally, thereby decreasing the body weight on the head, shoulders, and upper trunk. By the fifth month, the beginning of lateral postural control is seen as the baby begins to shift weight sideways in prone and supine.

In addition to symmetrical postural activity in prone and supine, postural synergies in sitting begin to develop at four to five months. From one longitudinal study of infants two to five months of age, it appears that they develop their own preferred patterns of postural synergies for sitting, and that these patterns become consistent on an individual basis by the fifth month (Wollacott and Shumway-Cook 1990). When placed in sitting and released to sit alone, all subjects slumped forward. However, the anterior displacement of the trunk was greater in the two- to three-month-old infant, and postural responses were quite variable. In contrast, the four- to five-month-old infant demonstrated three distinct patterns of postural activity in the lumbar spine and hips. The muscle response patterns utilized were lumbar extensors/quadriceps femoris, lumbar extensors/hamstrings, and hamstrings/quadriceps femoris, with the last two patterns resulting in the least amount of trunk displacement. From three to five months, sitting requires less support as the infant learns to control the trunk, shoulders, and head in space with the pelvis and lower extremities forming the base of support. The baby plays with movement within the range of this base while supported externally by an adult or seated device. Constantly organizing the visual, proprioceptive, and vestibular input with muscle activity, the baby is preparing for independent sitting at six months.

Primitive reflexes are no longer dominant as postural reactions and postural control develop. As the infant begins to control many movements by five months, the Moro or startle reactions are seldom seen. Proximal stability also enables the development of isolated joint movements and midrange control. For example, the four-month-old baby flexes and extends the knee in prone while keeping the hip extended. In supine, the five-month-old baby wiggles the toes and feet while holding the legs in the air. This coordination is only beginning in these early months and continues to develop as the baby gains postural stability in other positions against gravity.

■ Gross Motor Development

Anatomical and Range of Motion Characteristics

Motions of the head and cervical spine become almost complete and are used in functional movement. As a result of weight shifting and extremity movements, lateral and rotational thoracic motions continue to increase. The entire neck and thorax lengthen as soft tissue elongates and joints are less compact. Decreased skin folds and more definition of muscle bulk are evident.

Primary spinal curves that exhibit a posterior convexity are present in the newborn infant in the thoracic and sacral-coccygeal areas. Secondary curves with an anterior convexity develop in the cervical and lumbar areas in order for the skeleton to accommodate to a vertical position. Providing greater mechanical stability from the joint structure and ligaments, this system produces a biomechanical advantage so that less muscle activity is required to maintain an upright posture. The cervical curve is seen by four months as the infant can hold the head erect and steady. Although developing in prone, extension of the lumbar spine is not used in the sitting position until ten to twelve months and is more consistently present once the baby is standing and walking independently.

In prone, the contour of the low back changes from relatively flat at birth to concave, the result of increased range of lumbar and lumbosacral extension (figure 4.4). The articulation of the sacrum with the fifth lumbar vertebra begins to develop an oblique angle, the lumbosacral or promontory angle, which contributes to the total range of extension in the lumbar area (figure 4.5). This angle measures approximately 30 degrees for optimal erect posture in the adult (Norkin and Levangie 1983).

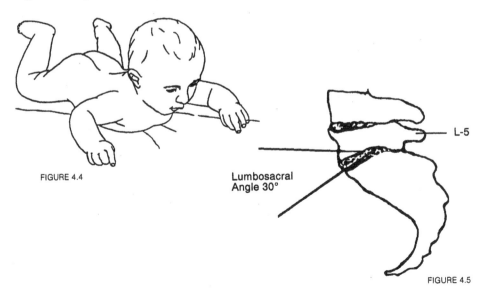

FIGURE 4.4

Lumbosacral
Angle 30°

L-5

FIGURE 4.5

The erector spinae, which are enclosed in the lumbo-dorsal fascia and the deeper multifidus, a large muscle that expands the entire vertebral column, have probably been active since birth as the infant moved in total extensor patterns. Now these muscles maintain sustained contractions for postural activity in prone and supine and, with ligaments, provide stability for the lumbar spine and the lumbosacral angle.

By the fourth to fifth month, the muscle bulk of the spinal extensors can easily be seen, forming a rounded vertical contour on the surface along each side of the lumbar spine and coming to a point at the most prominent portion of the sacrum (approximately the third sacral vertebra). A central furrow over the lumbar spinous processes and a triangular definition over the sacrum are evident. Dimples are seen over the posterior superior iliac spines of the pelvis, an important attachment site for muscle including the gluteus maximus, the origin of which is continuous with some of the erector spinae muscle fibers (figure 4.6).

In addition to spinal extension, hip extension is also increasing from three to five months of age. The gluteus maximus becomes extremely active and definition of the muscle bulk is clearly seen as the buttocks become rounded and firm. The development of spinal and hip extension allows the pelvis to lie parallel to the surface in prone (figure 4.6).

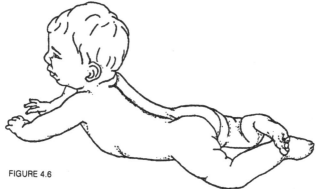

FIGURE 4.6

The joint capsule and other soft tissue surrounding the hip become more flexible. Active and passive ranges of hip abduction and the combination of flexion/abduction/external rotation increase as well as hip extension. The hamstrings elongate, resulting in a greater range of knee extension with the hip flexed. The capsular elements of the knee are also changing, indicated by more knee extension with the hip extended and reaching full range in many infants. Additionally, ankle plantar flexion and intrinsic foot mobility begin to increase. Although the mechanisms for these changes are not well understood, they are at least partially due to the infant's own active movement of the lower extremities.

Posture and Movement

Although stuck in whatever position placed in, the three-month-old baby appears to be content while learning to move body parts in limited ranges. The infant may even resist a change in position by arching the head and trunk or collapsing into a flexed posture. Some babies are quieter in their motor activity during the beginning of the third month. Less kicking and arm movements may be seen. Maturation of the central nervous system has reached a point where reflexive movements no longer dominate. Brain waves are changing and more closely resemble adult patterns (Caplan 1971). The baby now has some control over movements and can begin to repeat them just for the experience of moving. There is a time of disorganization as motor learning begins, but soon even the more passive infant experiments with movement of the whole body and of specific parts.

By the fifth month, an acceleration of motor activity is seen and continues throughout the first year as the baby learns to move and control the body in space. Displaying tremendous energy, the infant practices gross motor patterns repeatedly and often becomes frustrated if unable to transition from one position to another. Although some babies are less active in total body movements, they repeat other motor patterns such as sucking, reaching, and grasping toys, or playing with their fingers and feet (Caplan 1971).

Supine. Symmetrical postures and bilateral activity of the upper and lower extremities dominate during this time period. The three-month-old infant can hold the head in midline for long periods of time. Tucking the chin, the baby gazes downward toward the chest. This is flexion of the head on a stable cervical spine, a movement that can occur only if the neck is not in extension. The prevertebral neck muscles elongate or straighten the cervical spine, creating the proper biomechanical alignment so that bilateral action of the sternocleidomastoid muscle will flex the head. Stability of the trunk is provided by recruiting a total pattern of flexion, including activation of the pectorals, rectus abdominus, and the extremities. The upper extremities adduct across the chest and the hands grasp each other while the hips and knees flex, bringing the extremities closer to the center of the body mass (figure 4.7).

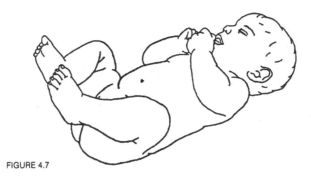

FIGURE 4.7

By five months, the infant has developed independent movement of the head and can tuck the chin without the total flexor synergy (figure 4.8). The infant can also lift the head in supine and might lift the shoulders off the surface, a sign of increased abdominal strength. However, it will be several years before the baby can independently sit straight up, an activity that requires greater hip flexor strength and stability of the pelvic girdle.

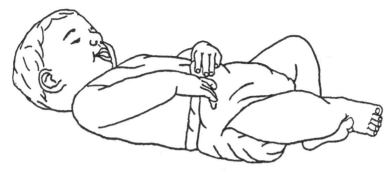

FIGURE 4.8

From three to five months, the infant continues reciprocal kicking of the lower extremities, although the movement differs slightly. Increased range of hip motion results in more abduction and external rotation of the femur as the hip flexes. Biomechanically this motion causes the pelvis to elevate laterally in the flexion phase of kicking and depress during the extension phase. Whereas the pelvis was pulled into the posterior/anterior direction at one to two months as the femur moved, now it is pulled in a different plane so that more lateral flexion of the lumbar spine occurs.

As postural stability of the trunk is developing, the baby improves in ability to lift and hold varying positions of the extremities against gravity. The three-month-old baby brings the arms across the chest, using grasp of the hands on each other or on clothes to maintain this position (figure 4.9). The baby also has the ability to bilaterally

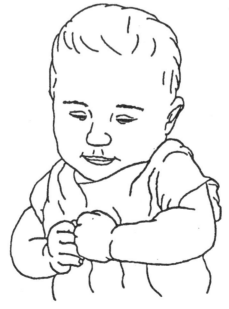

FIGURE 4.9

adduct the humeri and hold the forearm in a vertical position (figure 4.10). The baby can pull the knees up and symmetrically hold them for a short period of time, indicating a sustained contraction of the iliopsoas, which moves the femur into a pattern of flexion/abduction/external rotation.

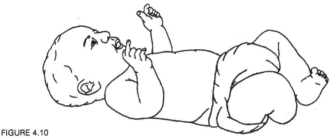

FIGURE 4.10

Whereas at three months trunk or pelvic movement is minimal during this activity, at four months, flexion of the trunk results in the pelvis tilting posteriorly, lifting the buttocks off the surface. Beginning to control forward flexion of the humerus against gravity, the infant reaches downward to touch the knee or thigh and may pull into more flexion using distal holding of the hands to increase proximal activity (figure 4.11). Abdominal musculature is strengthened by repetition of this movement, and the proximal portions of the hamstrings are elongated increasing hip joint mobility.

The five-month-old continues these same activities; however, the total flexion pattern of the trunk is no longer required, indicating a balance of flexor and extensor postural control (figure 4.12). A greater range of hip flexion/abduction/external rotation is possible and the infant now gets the hands to the feet while controlling the upper extremity with more elbow extension. The baby intently watches the feet and plays with the position of the lower leg in space as quadriceps activity begins to control the knee. The five-month-old baby also symmetrically lifts the legs in the air with knees extended and forcefully lowers them to the surface with a bang. This requires the hip flexors to stop contracting while the force of gravity acts on the lower extremities. The baby begins to control small ranges of hip movement while lifting one leg a few inches off the surface and maintaining the knee in extension then lowering it again.

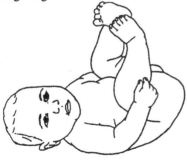

FIGURE 4.11

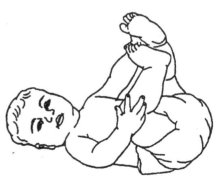

FIGURE 4.12

Not only do babies practice flexor activities against gravity in supine, but they also push back into extension against the surface, arching head, neck, and trunk. Repetition results in the infant pivoting or moving from one end of the crib to the other. Babies also use this extension pattern for communication (that is, letting a parent know when they are upset or do not like something). This extension, which occurs mostly in the upper trunk, is more asymmetrical at three months, resulting in rotation of the spine and a weight shift to one side (figure 4.13). The four-month-old infant begins to push with the feet while extending the hips, enabling the lumbar spine and lower extremities to be more active in the movement. The five-month-old infant adapts this pattern, lifting the pelvis while symmetrically extending the hips and maintaining the feet on the surface. This "bridging" activity requires that the head, shoulders, and upper trunk be stable (figure 4.14).

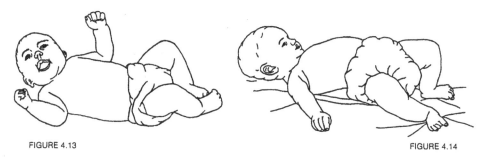

FIGURE 4.13   FIGURE 4.14

At about the fourth month, the baby lifts the legs and may lose symmetrical control. The pelvis falls to one side (figure 4.15). Spinal rotation occurs, resulting in elongation of the soft tissue posteriorly between the rib cage and pelvis, including the quadratus lumborum and latissimus dorsi musculature. Soon the baby begins to use the abdominal muscles, including obliques, to control some of the pelvic movement. Since body righting is present, the upper trunk may follow, and the baby rolls to a sidelying position. This first accidental rolling soon becomes fun, and the baby repeats it purposefully, staying on one side if the hands or an object catch the baby's attention (figure 4.16). Flexion of the underside hip blocks rolling to prone. Consequently, the baby cannot roll to the abdomen until the hip extends and the pelvis can rotate over the femur, usually not until five or six months of age.

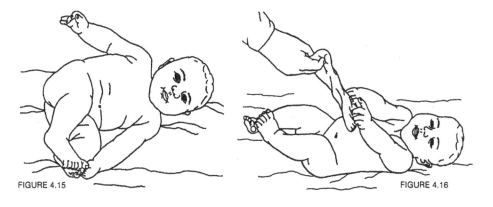

FIGURE 4.15   FIGURE 4.16

Prone. From three to five months, the infant's ability to lift the head and chest off the surface increases, and prone becomes a functional position. The upper extremities can be used for weight bearing and the lower trunk and legs provide stability for head and upper trunk activity.

At three months, the infant can symmetrically lift the head in prone, so the eyes are in a horizontal plane, shifting more body weight to the upper abdomen (figure 4.17). Positional stability is provided by the arms, which are more abducted and forward (elbows are in line with shoulder), and the flexed/abducted/externally rotated ("frog leg") position of the hips. Active stability is provided by the abdomen working off the surface, the spinal extensors, and probably some activity of the iliopsoas and gluteus maximus.

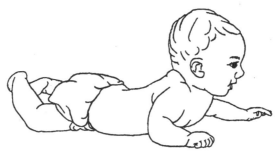

FIGURE 4.17

The four-month-old can prop on forearms, lifting the head and chest higher and shifting the center of gravity to mid abdomen (figure 4.18). Active stability increases with greater postural activity of the shoulder girdle and hip musculature as well as abdominals and spinal extensors, which now contract and hold more effectively. The infant can elongate the cervical spine, tuck the chin, and look down at the surface. In the fifth month, the baby pushes up to extended arms, shifting the center of gravity to the lower abdomen and thighs (figure 4.19).

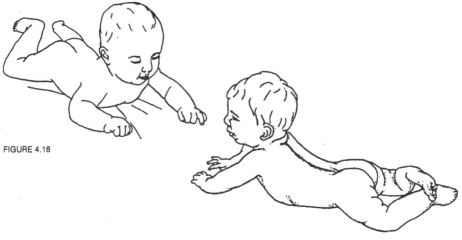

FIGURE 4.18

FIGURE 4.19

These new functional activities of the head, neck, upper extremities, and upper trunk require biomechanical changes to occur in the lower parts of the body. In addition to the general elongation of the thorax, hip mobility also increases. The increased abduction/external rotation of the hips at three months allows the pelvis to lower between the femurs so weight can be shifted from upper to lower parts of the thorax. The ability of the pelvis to lie parallel to the surface develops as more spinal and hip extension is available.

Although range of hip abduction/external rotation continues to increase, less external rotation of the hips is also used in prone, and a greater variety of lower extremity positions is seen. By five months, the baby can maintain a position of neutral hip rotation, lying with hips abducted and knees flexed or with adduction and knees extended. Since biomechanically these positions provide less stability against the surface, abductor activity (gluteus medius/minimus) along with extensor muscu-lature is required to stabilize the hip joint. Babies with lower postural tone tend to use the more extreme abducted/externally rotated position for a longer period, as it provides greater positional stability and requires less muscle activity.

From three to five months, the ability to weight shift in prone begins to develop. The three-month-old infant can turn the head in the vertical position, shifting weight over the shoulder on the face side (figure 4.20). By the fourth month, the weight shifts to the skull side, and prone head turning is now independent from the shoulder girdle (figure 4.21). By five months, the infant can shift weight to one arm using lateral and rotational control of the thorax and free the other for reach (figure 4.22). Initially, the

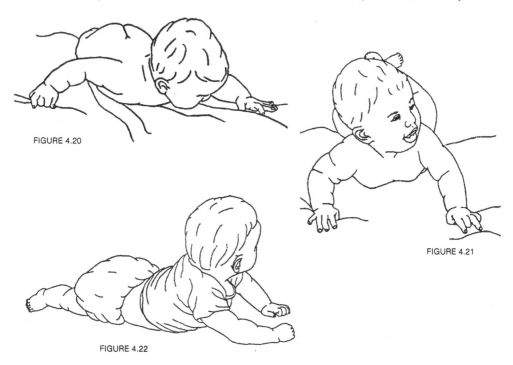

FIGURE 4.20

FIGURE 4.21

FIGURE 4.22

baby often shifts too far over the shoulder and, depending on the position of the humerus, accidentally rolls to supine. Unable to roll back to prone, the baby may fuss until someone places him on his abdomen. With repetition, the baby develops sufficient control of weight shift and does not lose balance while reaching in a variety of ranges.

During these months, the infant plays with movement in prone. The infant symmetrically extends the spine, lifting arms and legs off the surface. At four months, scapular adduction reinforces the thoracic extension; the elbows are flexed (figure 4.23). By five to six months, the arms can be held outstretched as greater strength and postural activity of shoulder girdle and anterior musculature (pectorals/abdominals) work with the spinal and hip extensors (figure 4.24). After this symmetrical bilateral activity begins, the baby extends the spine and moves the arms and legs reciprocally in a swimming motion. Asymmetrical movements may cause an uncontrolled weight shift in the lower trunk and pelvis resulting in accidentally rolling to sidelying or supine (figure 4.25).

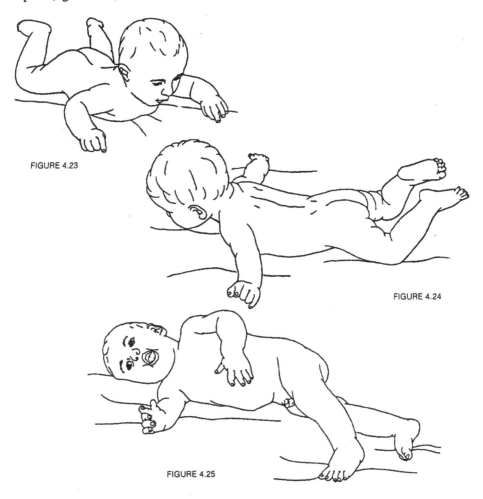

FIGURE 4.23

FIGURE 4.24

FIGURE 4.25

Babies practice these activities for long periods of time, developing balance, strength, coordination, and endurance as various subsystems develop and are uniquely organized within their movement system. The baby takes great pleasure in the vestibular and kinesthetic stimulation resulting from these movements, which are not only functional but also provide preparation for the development of other motor skills.

Sitting. By three months, the infant can hold the head upright in sitting, although support is needed around the thorax because postural control of the trunk has not yet developed sufficiently in an upright position (figure 4.26). Initially the spinal extensors activate from the lumbosacral area progressively upward, but the contractions are not sustained nor balanced by flexor activity. Consequently, the baby maintains an upright position briefly at first; however, the duration of holding rapidly increases throughout the month.

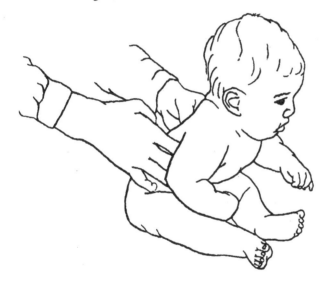

FIGURE 4.26

One of the most commonly available patterns that infants utilize to increase their stability or limit the degrees of freedom they need to control is shoulder elevation with humeral extension and elbow flexion. The pattern is frequently seen during the third month in sitting as the infant learns to control the head and trunk (see figure 4.26). The pelvis and lower extremities do not actively work off the surface and, therefore, do not provide an adequate base of support.

Babies this age sit upright infrequently, although they sit for long periods of time semi-reclined in an infant seat or swing. The back of the seat continues to function as a surface they can push against, providing stability for head and extremity movements. They may try to pull themselves to a more upright sitting position using abdominals, pectorals, and neck flexors, but cannot move their center of gravity forward over the hip joint. Motivated by visual stimulation, they play with their developing head control, lifting the head off the support, holding, and turning it.

The four-month-old sits upright for 10 to 15 minutes at a time, usually on someone's lap, and requires support only at the lower trunk or can now be held by the hands. This increased ability to sit upright indicates several developmental changes. Biomechanical aspects are altered as a greater range of hip external rotation/abduction is available, providing a more stable base of support. The upper extremity pattern of shoulder elevation, humeral extension, and elbow flexion is rarely seen in sitting as the infant can control a larger number of joints and joint motions. The secondary curve of the cervical spine develops for more efficient postural alignment of the head and neck, thereby decreasing muscle activity required to hold the head erect and steady (figure 4.27). Although extension has developed in prone, the lumbar spine is not held in an extended position in sitting until much later when the baby develops the ability to control the entire trunk in an upright position. Flexion of the thoracolumbar area helps maintain the center of gravity forward over the hip joint, a more stable mechanical position requiring less muscle activity and coordination. Practicing control of the body over the hips, the baby attempts to lean forward to reach or touch an object and return to an erect position. However, postural control has not developed sufficiently to prepare or support the movement so the adult holding the infant stabilizes the trunk or pelvis and assists the infant in coming back to upright. Therefore, sitting erect in a seat is not yet functional as the baby slides with attempts to move and reach.

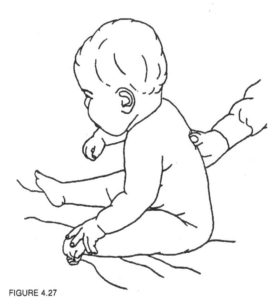

FIGURE 4.27

By five months, the hips externally rotate and abduct so the lateral side of the knees can almost touch the surface, providing a larger base of support. Biomechanically, a greater anterior displacement of the pelvis over the femurs is possible, bringing the center of gravity further forward with less rounding of the thoracolumbar spine. Consequently, the weight of the head, shoulders, and thorax stabilizes the femurs against the surface, and muscular activation around the hip joint acts on the pelvis, either moving it over the femurs or stabilizing it for movement above. The base of support is now more stable, allowing greater active control of the trunk. To limit the need to control the entire lower extremity and to provide distal stability, the feet often actively invert with flexion of the toes. Bringing the arms down and forward and requiring only minimal or intermittent support, the baby begins to prop on the hands. Sometimes the baby plays with the developing sitting balance, carefully trying to lift one hand to reach or play. At other times, the baby thrusts the body backward or leans far over to the side, challenging the responses of the adult holding the baby. Enjoying an upright view of the world, the baby uses the trunk and pelvic control to sit erect in a variety of seats, which include a bounce-type chair or walker, high chair, stroller, bath seat, and shopping cart. These give the infant different situations for learning to adapt postures and movements for functional activities; however, the infant is not safe and must be adequately secured and carefully supervised.

Standing. In addition to sitting erect, the infant's desire to be upright on the feet increases during this time period. The three-month-old baby may take weight only briefly, recruiting a total pattern of muscle activity in the lower extremities and requiring support of the trunk (figure 4.28). A wider base of support with greater abduction and external rotation of the hips provides more positional stability at four months (figure 4.29). The line of gravity passes anterior to the hip joint as flexion is

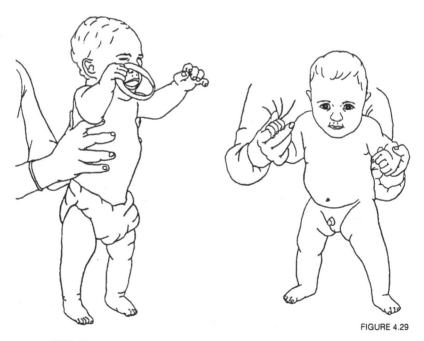

FIGURE 4.29

FIGURE 4.28

utilized to stabilize the pelvis over the lower extremities. Sufficient control to stand with the hip fully extended, as in the erect posture of the adult, does not develop for several years. However, the baby now has sufficient control to be held by the hands or forearms rather than supported at the trunk. Again the pattern of shoulder elevation with humeral extension and elbow flexion is used to provide stability for the head and trunk, similar to the pattern used in supported sitting at three months.

At five months, when pulled up from supine, the baby sometimes extends the legs and stands rather than sits. The baby also may pull up to standing from a sitting position when the hands are held, commonly seen when the baby is seated on an adult's lap, facing the adult. Continuing with the wide base of support, the baby may begin to let go, or stop the holding contraction of the quadriceps musculature, so the knees flex. Extending them again, the baby begins to control the knee in a weightbearing position. This beginning bouncing movement continues in the sixth month, providing vestibular, proprioceptive, and kinesthetic input in the upright position.

Development of the Feet

Starting at approximately the fourth month, the feet become more active in gross motor activities, developing isolated ankle motions and intrinsic movement. In supine with the legs held in space, dorsiflexion with inversion is seen without the total pattern of hip and knee flexion. As the infant kicks with a greater range of abduction/external rotation and extension/adduction, the plantar surface of the foot on the extending leg brushes along the inner surface of the opposite lower leg. This appears to stimulate plantar flexion with eversion and long toe extension, and perhaps it increases mobility of the multiple joints of the foot. While lifting the legs in supine, the five-month-old baby reaches for the feet, grabbing the toes and pulling them into extension. This helps elongate the long toe flexors and soft tissue surrounding the metatarsal heads. The feet touch each other and the baby plays with the toes of one foot with those of the other. These activities provide valuable tactile information to the bottom of the foot, which may be important for weight bearing.

Weight bearing on the feet in positions other than standing is an important part of the development of standing and walking. Beginning at three months, the infant can lie supine with hips and knees flexed and the feet supported on the surface. By five months, the feet actively push against the surface, providing distal stability as the infant lifts the hips in "bridging." The infant can also push the heel into the surface as dorsiflexion with inversion and toe extension occurs, a pattern similar to heel strike in gait. This distal fixing of the lower extremity may be used as the infant rolls from supine to sidelying with hip extension rather than flexion. Toe extension with plantar flexion also begins at five months as the infant pushes the toes into the surface in prone, similar to the pattern of pushing off with the toes when walking. However, in standing, the toes are still flexed, gripping the surface to provide distal stability.

■ Fine Motor Development

Anatomical/Structural Characteristics

The child between three and five months of age progressively develops functional control of the upper extremities in weight bearing and in reach. Initially the child learns to use the arms in a horizontal plane, or within a ninety-degree range.

Humeral abduction and adduction are the primary patterns of voluntary motion for the three- and four-month-old baby, both in prone and supine. Horizontal humeral abduction requires scapular adduction, which is a movement of the scapulae toward the spine. This horizontal motion also requires thoracic extension and a posterior movement of the clavicles (Kapandji 1982). Prior preparation of the shoulder girdle for this functional movement pattern took place in supine between birth and three months of age, as the infant randomly moved the body with scapulae and spine supported. The force of gravity helped expand the upper chest, lengthening anterior musculature, thus allowing the clavicles to move posteriorly (Boehme 1988). Random motion also created mobility within the gleno-humeral joints, giving the infant greater freedom of arm movement. The two-month-old infant began to experience active horizontal abduction with the asymmetrical tonic neck response. The three-, four-, and five-month-old child strengthens this pattern of motion as control of prone extension is developed.

Horizontal humeral adduction/flexion is a movement of the arms toward midline within a 90-degree plane. This movement requires scapular abduction, or movement of the scapula away from the spine. As the scapulae move away from the spine, the thoracic spine flexes slightly, and the clavicles move forward (Boehme 1988). The infant's early attempts to support the body and lift the head in prone help prepare the shoulders for this motion. At three and four months of age, the child strengthens the arms and shoulders by pushing symmetrically against the surface to raise the head higher and higher against gravity. By five months of age, the child has enough shoulder girdle strength to shift weight to one arm and reach out with the other.

The five-month-old child begins to move the arm above shoulder height due to new anatomical capabilities of the shoulder girdle. Humeral flexion as well as humeral abduction above the 90-degree plane require scapular upward rotation or movement of the inferior border of the scapula away from the spine and toward the axilla. Thoracic flexion and upward axial rotation of the clavicle are also required. The five-month-old baby, in prone, mobilizes the shoulder girdle during each accidental roll over an arm or each time the arm slides out from under the body as the baby's weight shifts. It is in the lack of postural control that the baby "accidently" or inadvertently gains more joint range and muscle and soft tissue length. All these changes prepare the baby for greater voluntary function.

The lower arm also gains in function between three and five months of age. Anatomically, the forearm attains greater freedom of motion as the child at four months laterally transfers body weight while propped on forearms. At the same time, this weight shifting lengthens the muscle and soft tissues in the radial aspect of the wrist.

As the four- or five-month-old begins to push up on extended arms, elbow and wrist flexors are lengthened. This collective input into the lower arm reduces the dominance of flexion, ulnar deviation, and pronation as the child reaches out to the world.

The hand benefits greatly from the proprioceptive input of weight bearing on extended arms. The palmar aspects of the hand expand in width and length as the child bears weight on it. Consequently, the transverse and longitudinal arches begin to develop, making it possible for the child to maintain a grip on an object and move the object around in space (Boehme 1988). The expansion at the heel of the hand also provides freedom of motion to the thumb. Consequently, the base of the thumb moves away from the palm and provides a point of stability for grasp. The child's ability to bring both hands to midline creates the possibility for hand-to-hand exploration, a prerequisite for object transfer and release. The child's capability for hand-to-mouth and hand-to-body contact helps to develop tactile awareness and discrimination in the hand.

Sensorimotor development is clearly a miraculous process of mastering what is now available and creating the potential for more advanced function. It is a whole body, whole system process. Curiosity, courage, and an enormous amount of energy drive the three- to five-month-old child to attain voluntary control of the body.

Upper Extremity Development

Between three and five months of age, the child experiences important proprioceptive and kinesthetic information through all aspects of the shoulder girdle and upper extremities. Critical experiences take place in the prone position where the arms are supporting and dynamically moving body weight. In addition, the upper extremities have an important influence on the development of the ribs, spine, pelvis, and legs. Conversely, the information that the upper extremities receive relies on the sequential development taking place in the rest of the body. For example, the three- to five-month-old child transfers body weight from the shoulders to the abdomen, pelvis, and femurs. This creates the potential for development of abdominal control. In turn, active abdominals provide stability of the shoulder girdle on the trunk, creating the possibility for dynamic control of the arms during reach and grasp. The interrelationship between gross motor and fine motor development is incredible and indivisible.

Prone. In prone, the three-month-old infant begins to use symmetrical arm and shoulder girdle activity against the supporting surface. The arms are abducted and elbows are now in line with shoulders on a horizontal plane. The infant uses symmetrical, horizontal, humeral adduction with internal rotation against the supporting surface to lift the head and chest (figures 4.30 and 4.31). This strengthens the sternal portion of the pectoralis major. As the scapulae abduct, the serratus anterior is activated, generating scapular stability on the rib cage. It requires significant effort to push the arms against the surface in this fashion and transfer body weight to the upper abdomen and femurs. Since the elbows are not yet positioned under the shoulders, the child cannot relax or sink into the position without a total collapse of the trunk and an unweighting of the lower body. The three-month-old

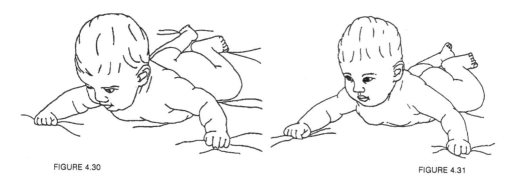

FIGURE 4.30   FIGURE 4.31

infant is driven by the desire to visually scan the environment. Therefore, the infant devotes tremendous energy in repeatedly pushing down with the arms to lift the head and chest. The infant may not want to stay in prone for long periods due to frustration and fatigue. At this age and in this position, the infant reaches out to the world with the mouth (figure 4.32). The shoulders and arms now provide adequate proximal control for this volitional movement of head, neck, and oral mechanism.

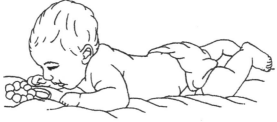

FIGURE 4.32

The four-month-old baby, in prone, begins to prop on forearms using the clavicular as well as the sternal portion of the pectoralis major. Consequently the arms push against the supporting surface with humeral adduction and flexion. This additional shoulder support reduces the effort required to function in prone. The anterior deltoid is also becoming stronger, giving the four-month-old baby greater shoulder girdle stability for dynamic control in prone.

The four-month-old baby begins to laterally shift the upper body weight. The baby does this by pushing off the supporting surface with one arm and transferring weight to the other arm (figure 4.33). Sometimes the supporting arm slides out from under

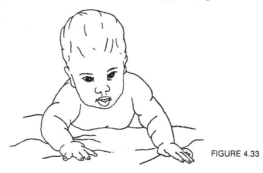

FIGURE 4.33

the body (figure 4.34) and the baby accidentally rolls over it. Rolling helps to lengthen musculature between the arm and the trunk, the humerus and the scapula, as well as the scapula and the rib cage. Ultimately, this elongation process generates ease of motion for reach in space.

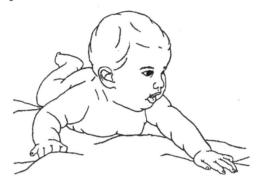

FIGURE 4.34

In prone, weight is often taken on the forearms and, during weight shifting, pronators and supinators are lengthened as the forearm rolls on the supporting surface. As the child shifts weight over the ulnar aspect of the forearm, radial deviation of the wrist is reinforced. As a result of this improved wrist alignment, the child moves to a more efficient grasp pattern.

The four-month-old baby also begins to push down with the hands, using partial extension of the elbows (figure 4.35). This weight bearing on the hands lengthens the long finger flexors as well as the intrinsic musculature and the soft tissue of the palm and thumb. This proprioceptive input to the palmar surface of the hand prepares the child for greater symmetry in grasp and the eventual participation of the thumb.

When presented with a toy, the child visually attends but does not yet have sufficient trunk control or shoulder-girdle strength to unweight one arm for reach. The child attempts to reach by using full body extension (figure 4.36). The child seems to be reaching with eyes and mouth as well.

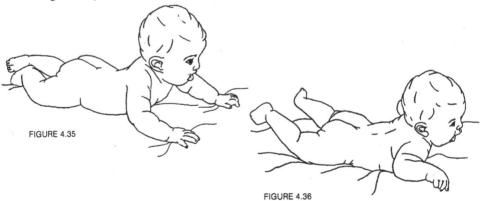

FIGURE 4.35

FIGURE 4.36

At five months, there is a dynamic change in the ability to interact with the environment in prone, since the child can now unweight an arm and reach out to the world. This new skill allows the child to develop isolated control of each shoulder girdle and arm, ultimately leading to a unilateral reach at six months of age.

At the beginning of the fifth month, the effort required to lift one arm and reach is so tremendous that there is difficulty maintaining eye contact with the object as the child moves (figure 4.37). By the end of the fifth month, the child has gained enough lateral and rotational control of the trunk to easily weight shift, reach, grasp, and play (figure 4.38). Due to increased deltoid and pectoralis major strength, the child can maintain the elbow in vertical alignment with the shoulder and trunk. The elbow is slightly forward of the shoulder, allowing for an unweighting of the hand and wrist.

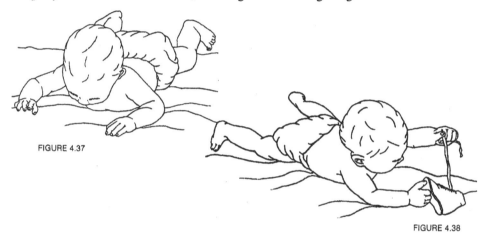

FIGURE 4.37

FIGURE 4.38

The child is able to laterally weight shift to the side of the arm and use both hands for exploration (figure 4.39). The weight-bearing arm is adducted against the trunk for stability. The child does have enough arm strength to abduct the humerus against the weight-bearing surface and return to a symmetrical prone position to continue with play (figure 4.40). Shoulder girdle depression has increased as abdominal control has developed. The child can rotate the forearms to neutral, putting both hands in a functional position for play. All aspects of the hand, including the thumb, are now fully opened due to the proprioceptive experiences received on the radial-palmar surface of the hand while in extended arm weight bearing.

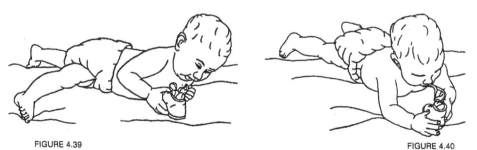

FIGURE 4.39

FIGURE 4.40

The child continues to gain in range of reach and, while in prone, can project the arm above the head (figure 4.41). This shoulder range is available because the lower spine is actively extended. The child cannot fully reach over the head in sitting until 11 months of age when active lumbar extension against gravity is developed.

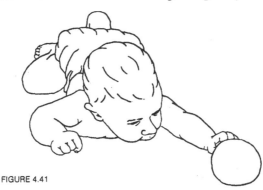

FIGURE 4.41

The child plays between prone extension and extended arm weight bearing. This is wonderful input for the shoulder girdle as it moves from scapular adduction with downward rotation (figure 4.42) to scapular abduction with upward rotation (figure 4.43). The child continues to increase strength in elbow extension. The child gains length in wrist extension and receives input that expands the hand in all directions. The balance developed between trunk flexion and extension creates proximal stability for reach in space as well as distal hand function in all positions. The child can support the body on extended arms in sitting. However, the protective extension responses needed to block a forward fall have not yet been developed.

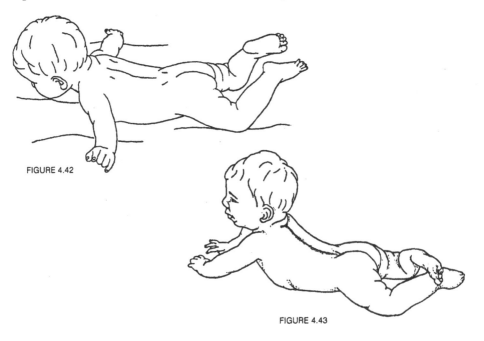

FIGURE 4.42

FIGURE 4.43

Supine. In supine, the three-month-old infant uses humeral adduction with internal rotation to bring the arms across the body. The infant can stabilize fisted hands against the chest (figure 4.44). The infant can press fisted hand against hand and bring both hands to the mouth (figure 4.45).

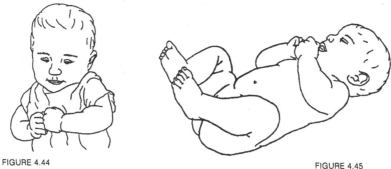

FIGURE 4.44   FIGURE 4.45

The ability to bring both arms into midline and to the mouth is due to the stability of the trunk as it recruits a total pattern of postural flexion. On the other hand, in supported sitting, the three-month-old infant brings the mouth down to the hands because in an anti-gravity position the infant lacks proximal control of the shoulder girdle and spine to lift the arms up toward the mouth (figure 4.46).

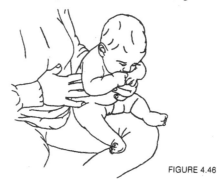

FIGURE 4.46

The three-month-old infant visually attends to objects. The infant may swipe at toys, symmetrically activating both arms, or may return to an asymmetrical movement pattern (figure 4.47). Arm motions are generally within an abduction and adduction plane and rarely move above 90 degrees. Elbows, wrists, and hands are flexed during swiping.

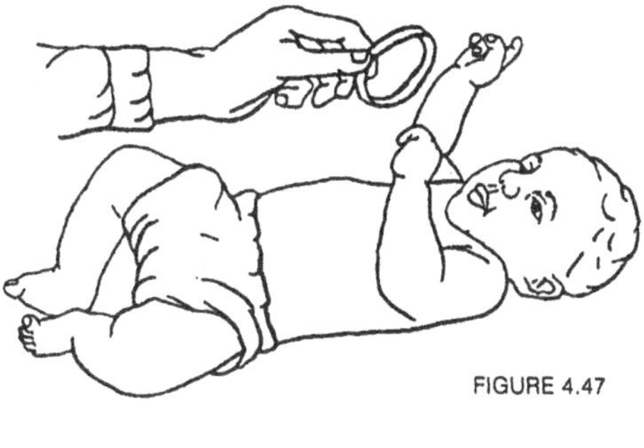

FIGURE 4.47

The four-month-old child uses a more consistent symmetrical approach to reach with elbows now extended to approximately 100 degrees (Erhardt 1982). There is less internal rotation of the humerus and the child is beginning to flex rather than solely adduct the arms (figure 4.48). Although still not able to reach above 90 degrees, the child can now briefly hold the arm in space while making contact with a toy. The four-month-old baby also continues to increase the range of hand-to-body contact and now can make contact with the head (figure 4.49) and thighs (figure 4.50).

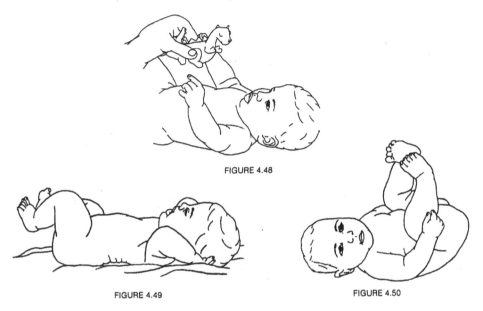

FIGURE 4.48

FIGURE 4.49

FIGURE 4.50

In supported sitting, the four-month-old baby reverts to the adduction pattern of reach and makes more consistent contact with toys (figure 4.51). Notice how the eyes, mouth, and arms are all reaching out to the toy. Like the three-month-old baby, this child brings the mouth down toward the toy for oral exploration (figure 4.52).

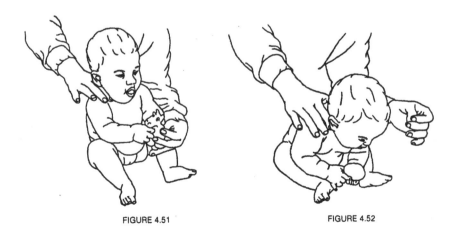

FIGURE 4.51

FIGURE 4.52

In supine, the five-month-old child continues to use a bilateral reaching pattern, but now one hand grasps the object first and then the other hand joins (figure 4.53). This is the subtle beginning of unilateral reach developed by six months of age. At five months the child can flex the humerus, rather than being limited to adduction. The elbows are extended to approximately 110 degrees (Erhardt 1982). The elbow flexors are progressively lengthened as the child plays hand-to-foot during the fifth and sixth months. The child at five months has great freedom of motion in the upper chest and arms (figure 4.54).

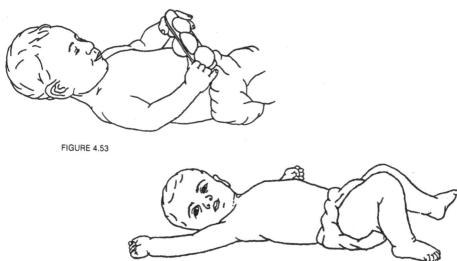

FIGURE 4.53

FIGURE 4.54

Hand Development

When the three-month-old infant's hand makes contact with an object, a sustained voluntary grasp is possible. The hand approaches the object with wrist flexion, ulnar deviation, and thumb adduction (figure 4.55). The ulnar digits are used for grasp (figure 4.56). The middle finger is the strongest, followed by the ring and little fingers (Erhardt 1982). The thumb is not active in the grasping process. The baby can maintain the grasp briefly and release is involuntary. At this age, the hand begins to accommodate or take the form of the object. The three-month-old baby scratches at clothing, body, and face, an indication that tactile awareness is developing in the hand.

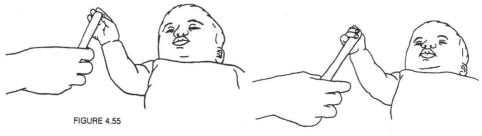

FIGURE 4.55

FIGURE 4.56

The hands of the four-month-old baby are generally opened as the baby approaches a desirable object (figure 4.57). The thumbs continue to be held in close proximity to the palm. There is variability in the grasping pattern of the child depending on the shape, size, and presentation of the toy (figures 4.58 and 4.59). The most consistent grasp pattern seen at this age is active flexion of the digits without involvement of the thumb. The wrist is less flexed than it was at three months. The child at four months does not yet have a voluntary release; however, mutual fingering in midline prepares the child to transfer objects from one hand to the other (Erhardt 1982). This activity is a precursor to controlled release in space.

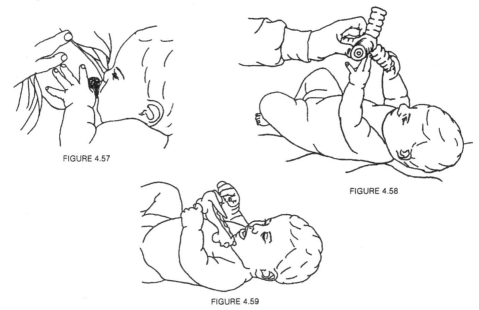

FIGURE 4.57

FIGURE 4.58

FIGURE 4.59

The five-month-old child is able to grasp an object with a symmetrical palmar grasp (figure 4.60). The fingers actively hold the object in the palm and against the base of the thumb. The distal portion of the thumb is adducted. The child's wrist position varies from flexion to neutral depending on the postural support provided to the trunk (figure 4.61). The less the proximal support, the more the child's wrist tends to flex for stability.

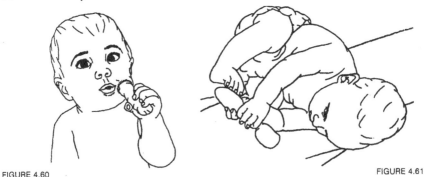

FIGURE 4.60

FIGURE 4.61

At this age, due to improved visual, tactile, and motor skills, the child makes more consistent contact with toys. The child now can easily bring the object to the mouth (figure 4.62), rather than bring the head down to the hands. Consequently, the child has enough proximal control to lift the arms up against gravity for finger feeding and oral and visual exploration. The child enjoys bringing the feet to the mouth as well. Now the child also shakes a toy using exclusively shoulder motions. The five-month-old child begins to explore objects due to the development of tactile discrimination in the hand (Erhardt 1982).

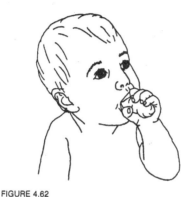

FIGURE 4.62

Continuing to develop preparation for a mature release, at five months, the child begins to transfer an object from one hand to another. However, it is effortful and slow. The child can release an object off the external stability provided by an adult holding or removing the object from the hand.

Visual Development

The midline orientation of the three-month-old infant, with developing symmetrical flexion, provides a proximal base of support for improved eye convergence, midline visual regard, and binocular fixation (Erhardt 1990). The baby observes the hand, a significant functional milestone. Eyes and head move together as the baby follows a horizontal moving target through a 180-degree range. This visual crossing of midline is still somewhat jerky at three months. The infant is able to shift glances between two objects, increasing the complexity of the visual world. The visual system is a strong incentive for the postural work that the infant initiates in all positions. The infant wants to reach out to the world that is now easily seen. Initially, the reach is with the eyes and mouth.

By four months of age, the baby is able to reach with the arms. It is a visually directed reach and grasp, supported by the increase in generalized anti-gravity postural control and the improved shoulder girdle stability developing in prone and supine. There is a delay between visual attention on an object and activation of reach and grasp. Sometimes the infant sees it and excitedly moves the whole body without reaching for the object at all. The range of the visual field now moves to the vertical and diagonal plane, expanding the visual world. The infant can visually fixate on nearby objects for longer periods of time. The infant can also briefly fixate on objects in further spatial fields (Erhardt 1990). Eyes begin to move independent of the head due to an increase in head and cervical control. There continues to be a midline jerk in visual tracking. However, the child can shift glances among three or more objects, but often temporarily loses visual fixation in the process.

The five-month-old child has more control of the body and subsequently better quality to visual control. This child now sees the object and immediately reaches for it. The eyes and hand have established a clear partnership. The child has improved horizontal, vertical, and circular eye tracking, can easily shift gazes, and can scan three or more objects with more consistent fixation (Erhardt 1990). This integrative period of visual system development prepares and entices the child to move around. The greater the child's visual field is, the greater the child's curiosity.

■ Oral-Motor and Respiratory Development

Anatomical/Structural Characteristics

Significant changes in the contour, shape, size, and alignment of the structures and musculature of the oral and pharyngeal mechanisms and the rib cage and diaphragm generally begin during four to six months of age, continuing on through puberty and into early adulthood. It is essential to recognize that many factors play a part in creating these changes in structure including genetic influences, growth and nutrition, and the active use of musculature for movement. Therefore, variations among individuals must be expected.

The following discussion of anatomical/structural characteristics is intended to provide a foundation of information in regard to changes that begin to occur in the normal infant as early as four to five months of age, but will take years until the process of anatomical change truly reaches what is recognized as characteristic of the adult population. It has been included in this chapter since many aspects of anatomical/structural change are difficult to pinpoint as to the specific months they can be noted within the first year of life. (A diagram of the adult oral and pharyngeal mechanisms is provided in Chapter 7.)

The oral and pharyngeal mechanisms. The skeletal framework of the oral mechanism undergoes significant changes as the oral cavity enlarges, the mandible becomes less mobile, the tongue and lips become more independent in their movements, and the teeth erupt. Development of the maxilla greatly influences modifications in the shape and alignment of the enlarging cavities of the mouth, nose, and orbits of the eyes.

The alveolar process of the maxilla enlarges as its bony element encloses the erupting teeth, creating a more distinctive delineation between the lingual and labiobuccal cavities within the oral mechanism. The shape and length of the alveolar arch changes in response to dental eruption, the size of individual teeth, and pressures placed upon the teeth from the tongue and lips. The palatine processes of the maxilla gradually increase in thickness and in bony composition with only slight transverse enlargement occurring primarily in its more posterior aspect. The greatest changes in the maxilla occur internally within its bony mass as the maxillary sinus expands it in a vertical dimension.

The hard palate, formed by the palatine processes of the maxilla and the palatine bones, changes extensively in its form from that of the newborn infant. Its growth in length occurs at its posterior (oral) aspect through the deposition of bone. The more deeply arched palate of the adult gradually develops over time in response to influences from oral and nasal cavity enlargement, alveolar arch contour changes, and tongue movements.

Growth of the palatine bones also involves increases in the vertical dimension that directly influences soft palate musculature attachments. The relationship between the hard and soft palates modifies as the musculature of the soft palate descends. This results in changes in the function of musculature such as the levator veli palatini, which now becomes more effective as an elevator of the soft palate during swallowing and sound production activities.

The mandible modifies extensively in its function as well as its size and shape. Although the mandible appears to grow in an anterior direction, the actual primary sites where growth occurs are posterior at the condyle and ramus (Ranly 1980). As the ramus enlarges, its shape also changes so that the condyle is angled in a more upward position. The angle between the ramus and body of the mandible will modify to approximately 138 degrees by two years of age, about 126 degrees by six years of age, and about 120 degrees in the adult (Bosma 1986).

The body of the mandible enlarges posteriorward to accommodate the increasing dental arch and along its lateral aspects to accommodate the tongue and need for greater space for chewing and biting activities. This is done through bone deposition occurring along its external aspects while resorption occurs along its internal aspects, modifying the shape of the body of the mandible. As was true for the maxilla, the alveolar processes of the mandible will enlarge and become firmer in composition as the teeth erupt.

Functional changes in the role of the mandible result as biting and chewing become more coordinated and as the temporomandibular joint modifies. The temporal fossa gradually deepens until a true articular eminence begins to be developed at approximately seven to nine years of age. The articular eminence will provide a more stable point for the mandible at the temporomandibular joint. This will reduce the overall mobility of the mandible while allowing it to become a more stable skeletal structure from which musculature of the oral and pharyngeal mechanisms can work more efficiently.

The facial musculature related to cheek and lip activity modify in accordance with the gradual elongation of the face, enlargement of the nasal and oral cavities, and changes in the form and alignment of other skeletal structures of the oral mechanism. As the influences of the panniculus and buccal, or sucking, fat pads reduce with growth, greater activity from the musculature of the cheeks and lips can be developed.

The tongue grows in length as well as in its transverse and vertical dimensions. As it grows and changes in its range of activity, it has a significant influence on the contour of the hard palate and alveolar ridge of the maxilla in addition to the form and position of the mandible and hyoid bone.

Of particular importance to future developmental advances is the fact that the posterior third of the newborn infant's tongue begins to descend gradually at approximately four to six months of age to eventually become part of the anterior wall of the pharynx by approximately four years of age. As the tongue begins to modify in its position, it has a direct effect on not only the other structures and musculature of the oral mechanism, but also on the shape and alignment of the structures and musculature of the pharyngeal mechanism.

At four to six months of age the pharynx begins to elongate and its structures begin to descend within the pharyngeal tube. By about five years of age, the curved contour of the newborn infant's pharynx has modified to form an obtuse angle at its junction with the posterior walls of the nasopharynx and oropharynx. At puberty, the pharynx has achieved its more adult shape at almost a right angle to the mouth and floor of the nasal cavity (Crelin 1973).

Although the length of the adult pharynx is approximately three times that of the newborn, its position in relation to the cervical spine shows minimal change. While the inferior aspect of the newborn infant's pharynx is at about the level of the fourth or fifth cervical vertebra, the adult's pharynx extends to approximately the fifth or sixth cervical vertebra. This suggests a significant connection between elongation of the pharynx and growth of the cervical spine, which supports the concept that a relationship exists between changes in the orientation of the pharynx within the head and neck and the orientation of the skull and cervical vertebrae throughout the developmental process.

As the pharynx elongates and descends, the three pharyngeal constrictors elongate and thin out as they cover the enlarging pharyngeal wall. This results in greater distinction between the musculature of the constrictors in the posterior wall of the pharynx as well as greater separation between the thyropharyngeus and cricopharyngeus, which compose the inferior pharyngeal constrictor. The internal longitudinal muscles of the pharyngeal wall also elongate during this process, becoming more active in pharyngeal shortening and constriction in conjunction with soft palate musculature activity.

As the posterior aspect of the tongue begins to descend and the pharynx begins to descend and elongate, the alignment of the structures and musculature of the pharyngeal cavity begins to dramatically change. The pharyngeal openings to the eustachian tubes begin to shift upward and backward during the first year of life until they reach a more adult-like position in the nasopharynx by approximately six years of age. The positional, internal stability provided by the close approximation of the tongue to the hard palate, soft palate, and epiglottis noted in the newborn infant will no longer exist, requiring the development of more mature musculature activity to successfully coordinate movements of the soft palate, tongue, epiglottis, hyoid bone, pharyngeal wall, and larynx during feeding, swallowing, and sound production activities.

The epiglottis gradually descends from its high position in the newborn infant to its position in the adult where its upper border is approximately at the level of the lower third or upper fourth cervical vertebra (Crelin 1973). According to Klock and Beckwith (1986), the epiglottis of the newborn infant, often described as omega-shaped or C-shaped, increases in its curvature during the first three years of life since growth appears to occur primarily in its sagittal diameter or anterior-posterior plane (length). It is not until after three years of age that the epiglottis begins to take on its more adult shape with a flattened contour as its transverse diameter (width) expands in size. As the epiglottis modifies in size, contour, and position, it projects into the pharyngeal cavity more than was noted in the infant. The depth and length of the valleculae increase as the spacial relationship between the epiglottis, posterior tongue, and lateral walls of the pharynx changes.

The hyoid bone descends from its elevated position in close approximation with the inferior border of the body of the mandible in the newborn infant to a more inferior position below the body of the mandible. As the larynx descends and its thyroid cartilage enlarges in the vertical dimension, the close approximation of the body of the hyoid bone and the thyroid cartilage noted in the infant modifies significantly. The hyoid bone becomes more angled in its orientation within the pharyngeal mechanism when compared to its alignment in the infant.

Changes in the contour, positional alignment, and function of the hyoid bone are greatly influenced by its musculature attachments (suprahyoids and infrahyoids) and through them, its direct association with the mandible, tongue, styloid process, larynx, shoulder girdle, and upper rib cage. As greater head, neck, shoulder girdle, and rib cage activity and postural control develop, the musculature attached to the hyoid bone from these structures directly impacts on the alignment and function of the hyoid bone. Reciprocally, the hyoid bone influences the development of controlled head flexion and neck elongation as well as shoulder girdle and rib cage activity. (See Chapter 8 for additional information on the larynx.)

As contour, shape, size, and alignment changes of the structures and musculature of the oral and pharyngeal mechanisms gradually occur, the infant learns to integrate and incorporate these changes into functional activities such as feeding, swallowing, and sound production. Structural changes begin early, but take years to be fully organized and coordinated for mature oral and pharyngeal function.

Rib cage and diaphragm. The contour of the rib cage modifies dramatically from three to five months of age as the ribs begin to angle downward and the rib cage begins to descend from the elevated position of the newborn. By five months, the rib cage exhibits a flatter overall contour.

The new antigravity movements of the infant during this time period have a direct impact on the rib cage, modifying its contour and alignment. The most significant of these influences on the rib cage include the following:

1. The infant is placed in supported sitting or standing, allowing gravity to passively pull downward on the ribs, sternum, and rib cage musculature.

2. More active spinal extension and greater mobility between the ribs and spine develop, especially in prone, as the infant lifts the head and shifts the weight back toward the lower rib cage and abdomen. This provides inward and downward input to the anterior rib cage.

3. Abdominal musculature (for example, rectus abdominus) begins to actively pull and hold the rib cage down, especially during supine and prone activities as well as during sound production. This provides a new active point of stability for the lower rib cage.

4. Elongation of the musculature and other soft tissue of the neck, shoulder girdle, thoracic area, and between the rib cage and pelvis frees the structures of the rib cage and the diaphragm for greater movement and changes in alignment. This prepares the upper rib cage for expansion during inhalation in the future.

5. New experiences with rolling and sidelying provide input to the lateral aspects of the ribs, to the musculature between the spine and ribs, and to the musculature between the ribs themselves. This assists in elongating soft tissue and preparing the rib cage for greater movement.

As the trunk elongates and the rib cage descends, the diaphragm moves downward from its higher position in the thoracic cavity, where it was in the newborn at rest. Since the musculature of the diaphragm is attached to the rib cage and upper lumbar vertebrae, movement of the diaphragm on inhalation will modify as greater lumbar extension develops and as the rib cage changes in contour and alignment.

Developmental Characteristics

The infant's use of the mouth to explore the environment steadily increases over the three- to five-month period. The mouth is used as the primary source for investigating toys or objects. This use of the oral mechanism is extremely important to the development of normal oral sensory awareness. It also provides new and different experiences in which the infant learns to move the structures of the mouth in conjunction with breathing and other body movements.

Infants now begin to experience a greater variety of oral-pharyngeal activity in relationship to the new general movement activities they are learning to accomplish. When tucking the chin in supine, the infant may experience a more closed-mouth position especially in regard to the jaw and lips (figure 4.63). As the infant plays in prone at four months of age, new lip movement and lip postures are often experienced in accordance with head and body movements against gravity (figure 4.64). When the infant is put in sitting (figure 4.65) or standing (figure 4.66), the lips, jaw, and tongue are often used positionally to provide and reinforce stability at the head, neck, shoulder girdle, and upper trunk. Through these new oral-motor experiences, the infant learns to coordinate oral and pharyngeal mechanisms with head, neck, and body movements and experiences new musculature activity that influences structural changes as well as functional movements.

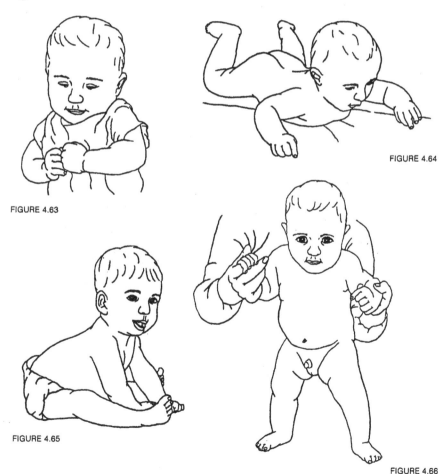

FIGURE 4.63

FIGURE 4.64

FIGURE 4.65

FIGURE 4.66

The feeding process. Although the forward/backward tongue movements and large, rhythmical up/down jaw movements characteristic of suckling continue to be predominant from three to five months of age, significant changes in oral movements gradually appear during this time period. Factors that directly influence these changes in oral function include the growth and new alignment of structures within the oral and pharyngeal mechanisms, the development of active head flexion and neck elongation, greater midline head orientation, increased active shoulder girdle stability, experiences with new food textures, and the development of new active oral musculature activity.

During bottledrinking and breastfeeding, the three-month-old infant exhibits increased voluntary control of the suckling process (Morris and Klein 1987). Greater cupping of the tongue to hold around the nipple may be used. Since the lips remain inactive, liquid is lost from the center and corners of the lips. Coughing, choking, and gagging continue to occur at times. The rooting response, automatic phasic bite-release pattern, and the gag response still influence the feeding process.

At approximately four months of age, the infant begins to modify the suckling movements used during bottledrinking and breastfeeding. The center portions of the upper and lower lips begin to actively hold on the nipple, providing a new active point of stability for the oral mechanism (figure 4.67). Although the jaw continues to move primarily in an up/down direction, the size of its vertical excursions is more limited due to the new lower lip activity. The tongue cups around the nipple and begins to exhibit greater up/down movements in response to the new oral stability provided by the lips, the more limited range of up/down movements of the jaw, and the structural changes starting to occur in the oral mechanism which provide greater intra-oral space for its up/down movements. These new oral movements in conjunction with the initiation of anatomical changes and neurological maturation mark the beginnings of the infant's transition from the immature oral movements of suckling to the development of mature sucking activity for bottledrinking and breastfeeding. Liquid loss is still evident, especially from the corners of the lips since the cheek and lip musculature in this area is not yet active.

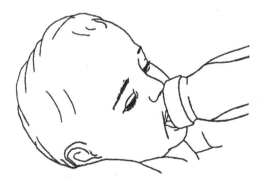

FIGURE 4.67

In the fifth month, the infant is gaining experience in using the new oral activity during bottledrinking and breastfeeding. Voluntary control is increasing as responses to stimulation that had elicited the rooting response and automatic phasic bite-release pattern diminish. The infant visually recognizes the bottle or breast, opening and quieting the mouth in anticipation of nipple insertion.

Although some infants are given baby cereal in the first few months of life, the presentation of semisolids, generally, is not encouraged until four to six months. At this time, the infant has greater oral-pharyngeal activity for handling semisolids by spoon and the gastrointestinal system has matured to a level to allow for better digestion of the food with less potential for allergic reactions (Pipes 1981; Robinson et al. 1986). However, the parents' decision to introduce semisolids is often not based on scientific data, but rather on the advice of family members and friends or the parents' perception that the baby is hungry and ready for food.

When an infant is initially given semisolids by spoon, a suckle pattern is used. Suckling movements are initiated as the spoon touches the lips. Although the lips may show some forward posturing, they are not active during the spoonfeeding process. Therefore, food is scraped off on the upper gums or upper lip by the feeder (figure 4.68).

Most pureed food that enters the mouth is pushed out due to the forward/backward movements of the tongue and the lack of lip activity. The small amount of food that remains in the mouth is moved back with the tongue movements. It is finally swallowed using tongue protrusion as a way of stabilizing the tongue in a more forward position so the food can be cleared out from the oropharyngeal area (figure 4.69). The feeder scrapes off food that is left on the infant's lips or chin and puts it back in the mouth, continuing this process until most of the initial spoonful has been eaten.

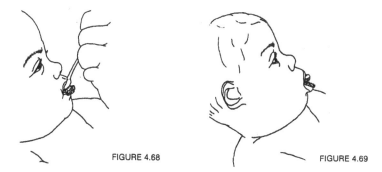

FIGURE 4.68   FIGURE 4.69

Since the infant has a fairly strong gag response, the introduction of a new texture like semisolids results in some gagging when the food reaches the back part of the tongue. As the infant continues to receive semisolids by spoon, the gag soon becomes more integrated in regard to this new texture. Each time a new, unknown texture is introduced to an infant, a gag response can be expected for a short period of time.

Teething may begin at approximately five months of age. In response to the swelling of the gums during teething, the infant sucks or "bites" on the fingers or other objects to help alleviate some of the discomfort. To help soothe the baby and in anticipation of teeth eruption, parents often introduce solids such as hard teething biscuits at this time.

This is the infant's introduction to solid foods. The infant scrapes this hard-type of solid on the gums, uses phasic up/down movements of the jaw that are not powerful enough to actually bite through the solid, or suck or suckle on the solid, especially if it is placed in the center of the mouth (figures 4.70, 4.71, and 4.72). As the infant's saliva softens the solid, small pieces may come off, which the infant usually spits out (figure 4.73). If a piece falls to the back of the tongue, the infant gags or chokes on it before spitting it out or swallowing it whole. Parents must stay close and watch the baby carefully whenever solids are given so that too large a piece does not break off and create problems.

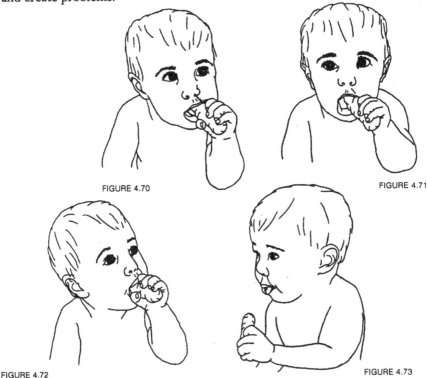

FIGURE 4.70   FIGURE 4.71

FIGURE 4.72   FIGURE 4.73

Occasionally parents give the five-month-old infant a softer solid such as a cookie or cracker. Although phasic up/down jaw movements are used on the cookie as it is placed on the biting surfaces of the gums, the infant cannot bite through it. The infant often attempts to suck or suckle on it. As was true for the hard-type of solid, saliva mixes with the soft solid so that pieces break off to be spit out or swallowed whole. These early experiences with solids lead to the early chewing and biting activities that will be developing at six months.

As infants begin to receive semisolids by spoon, they are often placed in a semi-reclined infant seat for feeding. This provides them with the stability and alignment they require at the head, neck, and trunk to allow them to more actively use the mouth for spoonfeeding. When infants are initially presented with solids, they are often held fully supported on an adult's lap so as to provide maximal body stability and safety. Soon the infant has sufficient head, neck, and body control to be placed in a high chair for some feeding activities.

Significant components of respiratory function. The infant's respiratory pattern at three to five months continues to be characterized by belly breathing. The contour and alignment of the rib cage is changing so that it appears flatter in contour. Lower rib expansion or rib flaring on inhalation may be more evident especially when the infant is in supine (figure 4.74).

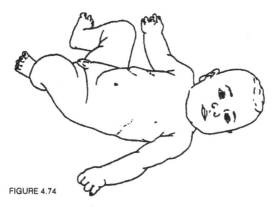

FIGURE 4.74

As greater thoracic spinal extension, lumbar spinal extension, hip extension, and abdominal musculature activity develop at five months, the depth of the infant's belly-breathing pattern starts to modify. On inhalation, greater belly expansion may be evident, although the rib cage exhibits minimal movement except at the lower ribs. Longer sounds are produced with more variety in their loudness and intonation patterns. Sounds appear less nasal in quality.

When actively moving in a position like supine or prone, periods of asynchrony in the rhythm of the infant's breathing may occur. This is probably associated with the infant's inability to smoothly coordinate new musculature activity being learned in general movement with a changing respiratory mechanism. As new movement patterns are repeated and integrated by the infant, respiratory function with movement becomes more coordinated.

Sounds continue to be produced with body movement and are modifying in accordance with the new body and oral movements the infant is experiencing in different positions. The lips seem to influence sound production in prone, while tongue and jaw movements appear to impact more on sounds produced in supported sitting. When in supine, sounds have a throaty quality with more posterior tongue activity involved in their production.

Summary Chart–3-5 Months

Postural Control	Gross Motor	Reach	Fine Motor
Head righting reactions developed; functional head control in all positions	*Increased range of motion* • full range of cervical motion, cervical curve present • thoracic and lumbar-sacral extension • thoracic lateral and rotational motions • hip extension, abduction, flexion/abduction/external rotation • full range of knee extension • plantar flexion	Voluntary swiping and reaching	Sustained voluntary grasp replaces grasp reflex
Trunk righting when tipped forward and backward in space; lateral righting beginning in fifth month	*Supine* • tucks chin (3 months); lifts head (5 months) • lifts, holds and moves limbs in space • hands to knees (4 months), hands to feet, (5 months) • "bridges" (5 months) • rolls to side (4-5 months)	Range of reach varies with position and degree of support	Uses fingers in grasp without thumb involvement at 3 months
Landau reaction begins at 4 months, complete at 5-6 months		Begins to reach forward	Progresses to symmetrical palmar grasp at 5 months
Develops antigravity flexor and extensor activity in supine and prone, respectively	*Prone* • lifts and holds head erect • props on forearms (4 months) • pushes up on extended arms (5 months) • lifts arms and legs off surface (4-5 months) • swimming movements (4-5 months) • accidentally rolls to supine (4-5 months).	Bilateral reaching pattern	Hand begins to accommodate to the shape of an object
Maintains symmetrical postures		Strong hand-to-mouth pattern	Tactile awareness develops in the hand
Weight shifts laterally through head, shoulders and upper trunk	*Sitting* • sits upright for brief periods with upper trunk support (3 months) • sits upright 10-15 minutes with lower trunk support (4 months) • props on arms in sitting with minimal or intermittent support (5 months) • sits erect in a variety of seats; needs safety strap (5 months)		Begins to transfer hand to hand
Beginning of postural activity to prepare for and support volitional movements	*Standing* • stands with arms or hands held and wide base of support (4-5 months) • may begin to bilaterally flex and extend knees (5 months)		*Some infants develop activities earlier or later than this chart indicates. Therefore, it should not be regarded as a rigid timetable of events.*

Summary Chart–3-5 Months continued

Vision	Oral-Motor/Feeding	Respiration-Phonation
Binocular fixation	Rooting response and automatic phasic bite-release pattern diminishing	*Respiration* No longer an obligatory nose breather as oral-pharyngeal structural alignment begins to modify
Eye convergence	Strong gag response; begins to diminish at about 5 months	
Visually crosses midline	*Feeding* Shows more voluntary control of mouth during bottledrinking/breastfeeding	Belly breathing with flatter anterior rib cage contour is predominant; deeper inhalation may begin by 5 months
Vertical and diagonal visual tracking	• uses center portions of lips to hold on to nipple at 4 months • uses more active sucking with suckling by 5 months • liquid loss from lip corners	Periods of asynchronous breathing rhythm may occur with active movement, excitement, and effort
	If spoonfeeding, uses suckling; gags on new textures	*Phonation/Sounds* Produces different cries for pain, anger, fussing, hunger, and in connection with different people
	May begin to receive solids at 5 months • scrapes hard solids on gums • uses phasic, up/down jaw movements, suckling, and sucking on soft/hard solids • if piece of solid falls back on the tongue, will gag and then spit it out or swallow it whole	Vocalizes more; cries less
	Oral-Motor Uses mouth to explore objects in environment	Coos with greater variety of consonant sounds, longer duration, and less nasality by 4 months
	Experiences new oral movements in association with developing head and body control/movements	Produces greater variety of vowels and consonants with new mouth and body movements; begins babbling at 4 months
	Drooling decreases in positions with greater postural stability; may increase with teething	

■ References

Boehme, R. 1988. *Improving upper body control*. Tucson, AZ: Therapy Skill Builders.

Bosma, J. F. 1986. *Anatomy of the infant head*. Baltimore: The Johns Hopkins University Press.

Caplan, F. 1971. *The first twelve months of life*. New York: Grosset and Dunlap.

Crelin, E. S. 1973. *Functional anatomy of the newborn*. New Haven, CT: Yale University Press.

Erhardt, R. P. 1982. *Developmental hand dysfunction*. Tucson, AZ: Therapy Skill Builders.

Erhardt, R. P. 1990. *Developmental visual dysfunction*. Tucson, AZ: Therapy Skill Builders.

Kapandji, I. 1982. Upper limb. In *The physiology of the joints*, Vol. 1. New York: Churchill Livingstone.

Klock, L., and J. B. Beckwith. 1986. Appendix: Dimensions of the human larynx during infancy and childhood. In *Anatomy of the infant head*, edited by J. F. Bosma, 368-77. Baltimore: The Johns Hopkins University Press.

Morris, S. E., and M. D. Klein. 1987. *Pre-Feeding skills*. Tucson, AZ: Therapy Skill Builders.

Norkin, C., and P. Levangie. 1983. *Joint structure and function*. Philadelphia: F. A. Davis.

Pipes, P. L. 1981. *Nutrition in infancy and childhood*. St. Louis, MO: C. V. Mosby.

Ranly, D. M. 1980. *A synopsis of craniofacial growth*. New York: Appleton-Century-Crofts.

Robinson, C. H., M. R. Lawler, W. L. Chenoweth, and A. E. Garwick. 1986. *Normal and therapeutic nutrition*. New York: Macmillan.

Wollacott, M. H., and A. Shumway-Cook. 1990. Changes in postural control across the life span—a systems approach. *Physical Therapy* 70:799-807.

Chapter 5

6 Months

■ Postural Control

By six months of age, the baby has sufficient postural tone to maintain many postures against gravity. The baby sits for long periods of time, stands tall with hands held, and actively holds a variety of other postures in supine, prone, and sidelying. There is greater postural activity of the lower trunk, pelvic girdle, and lower extremities than in previous months. The baby can now shift the weight from the lower part of the body in supine, prone, and sidelying, working off the supporting surface. This provides more lateral control and allows greater dissociation of one side of the body from the other. These postural responses are used to accompany focal movements, such as reach, or to transition the body in space, as in rolling. The baby controls forward and backward movement of the center of gravity in sitting and begins lateral control; however, arm support is needed for most ranges of weight shift.

By six months, labyrinthine and optical righting have fully developed. When the baby is held upright and tipped in space, head and trunk righting reactions are elicited in forward, backward, and lateral directions. The upper and lower extremities are often active in the response, flexing bilaterally when tipped back, extending bilaterally when tipped forward, and flexing unilaterally on the shortened side when tipped sideways (figure 5.1). In the horizontal position, a mature Landau reaction is present with hip and knee extension; abdominal activity balances the extensor activity to enable an elongated holding posture of the trunk.

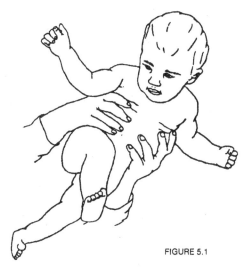

FIGURE 5.1

Forward protective extension of the arms, another postural reaction, begins to emerge at six months. When held in space and tipped forward to the surface, the infant catches himself or herself with extended arms. In addition, equilibrium reactions are present in prone and are beginning to be seen in supine. A mature body-on-body righting response can be also elicited. When the head is passively turned in supine, rotation occurs progressively down the spine resulting in the body segmentally following the movement of the head. Previous to this time, the trunk moved as a total unit without spinal rotation.

■ Gross Motor Development

Supine. The six-month-old baby demonstrates greater anti-gravity motor control in supine, indicating increased strength, endurance, and coordination of patterns as well as improved postural activity. The baby can raise one or both arms freely in space and reaches to be picked up. The baby also lifts the legs in the air without rolling the pelvis, signifying greater freedom of leg movements from a stable pelvic girdle (figure 5.2). This is in contrast to the five-month-old infant who used a shortened contraction of the rectus abdominus to tilt the pelvis posteriorly while lifting the legs. Increased mobility into hip flexion may also account for the ability to further move the femur without accompanying pelvic motion. Both increased flexibility of the posterior aspect of the joint capsule and the proximal end of the hamstring musculature probably contribute to this mobility. Many six-month-old babies have the ability to hold their legs vertical with the knees extended, indicating not only greater control, but also increased length of the distal hamstrings. They continue to play with their feet and are frequently in motion, arching and twisting the trunk, reaching, bridging, moving their legs, and rolling over. This makes dressing and changing diapers exasperating for parents!

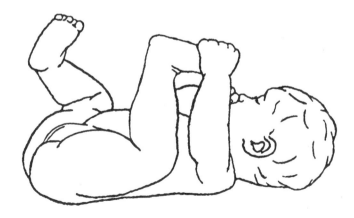

FIGURE 5.2

Sidelying. Although the four- to five-month-old infant was able to maintain sidelying briefly, the six-month-old can now stay in this position for longer periods. As the baby reaches and plays, postural activity and other aspects of motor control have developed sufficiently to allow a variety of postures and movements. The infant reaches in a greater range without losing balance and falling to prone or supine. Lower extremity dissociation is now possible in this position as one leg can be extended and the other flexed. The baby reaches and plays with the feet (figure 5.3) and may try to move or locomote to get a toy by pulling the body across the floor (figure 5.4). Distal stability can be provided by active contact of the foot with the surface. The lower leg and intrinsic musculature activate in various combinations, dependent on the relative alignment of the tibia over the foot. The motor control system receives tactile and proprioceptive information about weight bearing on the medial or lateral aspects of the plantar surface, which may be important for postural activity of the foot in other positions in later development (figure 5.5).

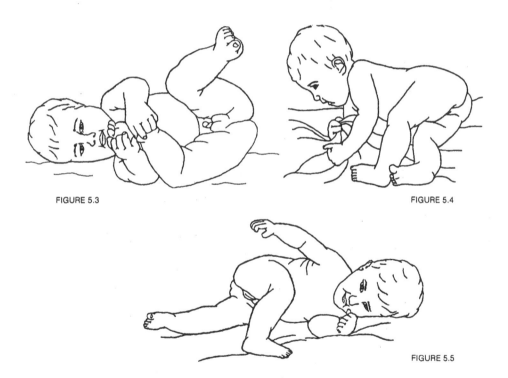

FIGURE 5.3

FIGURE 5.4

FIGURE 5.5

The desire to get upright can be observed as the baby tries to sit up from the sidelying position. The baby flexes the trunk, pulls with the arms, flexes the hips, and extends the knees. However, inability of the weight-bearing hip to push against the surface, insufficient strength, and lack of rotational control prevent raising of the upper body off the surface. The baby practices this in the months to come, but will not be able to complete the transition until ten to twelve months. To be successful, the baby learns to roll to prone and assume sitting from a quadruped position.

Prone. By the sixth month, prone becomes an important position for play as the infant now has sufficient postural stability to practice a greater variety of movement patterns while lying on the abdomen. Motor control improves in symmetrical and asymmetrical postures and the extremities are free to move in wide ranges on and off the surface.

Increased postural activity of the spinal extensors, oblique abdominals, and hip extensors allow the baby to hold an elongated horizontal position in prone (figure 5.6). Arms and legs outstretched, the baby attempts to reach for objects at arm's length. Quadriceps activity often accompanies the reach as well as dorsiflexion or plantar flexion of the feet, providing distal stability for the forward movement of the arm.

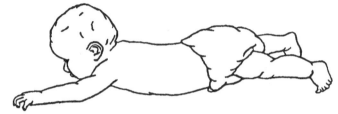

FIGURE 5.6

The six-month-old child experiments with more movement of the trunk in prone. The child moves it laterally, often extending or elongating the side that is shifting, and flexing or shortening the opposite side. This pattern at six months differs from the one that occurred at five months in that the weight is now shifted through movement of the lower thorax and pelvic girdle rather than through the upper trunk and shoulder girdle. This provides more efficient biomechanics and stability for upper and lower extremity movement in a wider range. The baby experiments with how far the weight is shifted and gains control of moving through the space between prone and sidelying (figure 5.7). Upper extremity postures include various combinations of weight bearing on forearms and extended arms, and the arm on the shortened side is capable of moving through space (figure 5.8). Lower extremity positions also vary with more options for movement available. The pattern of one leg extended (elongated side) with the other flexed (shortened side) signifies dissociation of one leg from the other and prepares for the reciprocal pattern used in belly crawling.

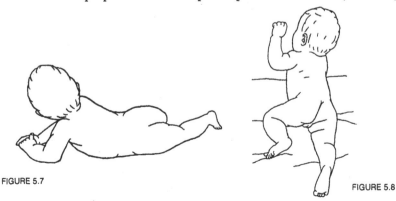

FIGURE 5.7

FIGURE 5.8

Pushing up to extended arms is easier for the baby now than it was at five months. The baby can lift the chest higher off the surface as upper extremity strength has increased and oblique abdominal musculature and hip activity provide greater stability caudally. Some babies can do this only with symmetrical lower extremities; however, babies with greater postural control may flex the hip and knee of one leg while holding the other extended, a pattern that can later be used to assume the quadruped position (figure 5.9).

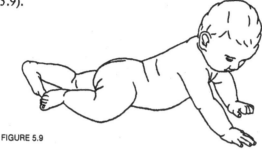

FIGURE 5.9

The instinctive need to be upright is strong and the six-month-old baby attempts to get up on hands and knees. When propping on forearms, the baby symmetrically pulls the knees up under the body and pushes down on the forearms, using synergistic activity of the pectoral muscles and abdominals. Pushing first on one hand and then the other, the baby works intensely to assume the quadruped position (figures 5.10a, b, c, d). Unable to coordinate postural activity of the hips, trunk, and shoulder girdle, the baby loses balance and falls forward. As motor control develops in relation to postural stability, muscle strength, and coordination, repeated efforts result in the baby shifting the center of gravity backward by moving the pelvis over the knees. Most babies learn to maintain quadruped between six and seven months of age.

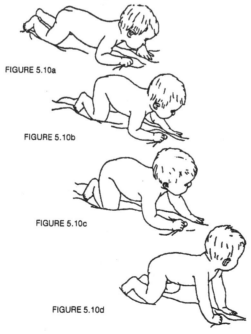

FIGURE 5.10a

FIGURE 5.10b

FIGURE 5.10c

FIGURE 5.10d

The infant's desire to locomote is beginning to appear at this time. When on forearms and knees, an active baby may lunge forward while spreading out the arms and legs. Returning to the forearm/knee position, the baby repeats the forward weight shift and may move a few feet across the room. Some babies also begin to push themselves backwards from this position. Although most six-month-old babies cannot efficiently belly crawl or pivot, they may try to pull themselves forward or sideways if they can grasp a stable object, for example a crib rail, an adult's hand, or even a blanket.

Rolling. Most babies can transition between supine, prone, and sidelying by the end of six months, and the first means of locomotion can be observed as the baby learns to consecutively roll across the bed or floor. As with all movement patterns, practice is required. Some babies take longer to develop this skill than others. Each baby develops an individual pattern for rolling that becomes more efficient with repetition and motor learning. Lying on the back, the baby may push with one foot, shifting weight from the heel to the forefoot as the ankle plantar flexes. Hip, knee, and spinal extension accompany the push off from the foot, shifting the body weight onto one side to the point where gravity favors prone (figure 5.11). The baby flexes the leg to bring it forward from a trailing position and extends it again to allow the pelvis to lie flat as the baby reaches prone. The upper extremity may follow the thorax, but needs to move into a position of forward flexion for efficient weight bearing in order to maintain head control as the shoulder girdle approaches the surface.

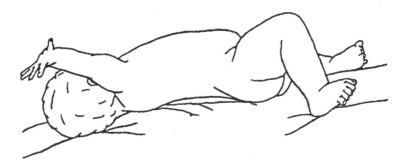

FIGURE 5.11

Another common rolling pattern consists of flexion of the hip and knee and horizontal adduction of the arm with flexion and rotation of the trunk to initiate the lateral weight shift in supine. The side the weight is shifted to is actively pushing against the surface for stability. As the baby approaches sidelying, elongation of the under side with lateral flexion of the upper side and abduction of the upper leg occurs for postural stability. As the arm and leg flex forward, extensor activity grades the movement to prone. The upper and lower extremities move into a functional position for prone during the terminal phase of the movement (figures 5.12a, b, c).

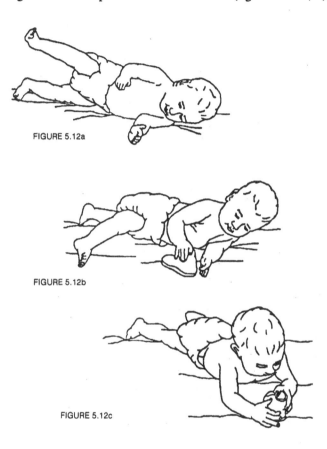

FIGURE 5.12a

FIGURE 5.12b

FIGURE 5.12c

One important component for rolling is hip joint mobility into internal rotation. As the pelvis moves over the fixed lower extremity on the weight-bearing side, the femur is relatively internally rotated. This is necessary for a graded movement into prone. Another important characteristic is that the weight-bearing side actively works against the surface as the body rotates around its axis, providing stability for the movement.

The six-month-old child has more control and coordination when rolling prone to supine than during the first accidental rolling at five months. The head and shoulders are higher off the surface because the baby can maintain and move the center of gravity from the lower trunk and pelvis. The baby sometimes stops at various points in the movement, indicating postural activity that is well developed and timed with the movement pattern. During this stage of development, the baby is gaining control of moving the body in a complete revolution around its axis in a horizontal plane.

Sitting. Although unable to assume the position independently, the six-month-old child pulls the body to sitting when an adult takes the hands. The baby enjoys this activity and practices it with each diaper change. Tucking the chin, the baby pulls with the arms, abdominals, and hip flexors and extends the knees while bringing the body weight forward.

By six months, the baby is able to sit well in a high chair and begin to control the limited surrounding space. The baby can lean on the chair or tray if the center of gravity moves too far, but quickly learns to bring the body back to an upright position to eat or play. Seated toys such as a spring horse with an infant seat or a jump seat are popular at this time because the baby enjoys pushing the feet against the surface and bouncing. Through these kinds of activities, the child learns control of whole body movements in a sitting position.

During this month most babies begin to sit independently on the floor with arm support and may easily play in this position for up to half an hour (Caplan 1971). Some are very steady and lift one or both arms for play; others may be wobbly and easily fall over with any weight shift. A cautious baby may move only slowly and in small ranges, developing postural control along with movement. Another baby may be motivated to experiment with development of other skills, although postural activity is not sufficient to support the movement. The baby explores and reaches for toys that are out of reach, developing perceptual and cognitive abilities, even though the movement is followed by a fall. Parents often place pillows around the six-month-old baby so the baby can play safely while learning to sit on the floor.

Most babies this age still require minimal support of the pelvis or lower portion of the trunk for ultimate function of the upper extremities in sitting (figure 5.13). Activities such as reaching forward in space and trying to manipulate or bring a toy

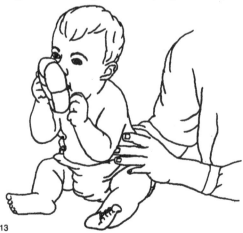

FIGURE 5.13

to the mouth require more postural control than most six-month-old babies have developed. Infants learn to be stable in sitting and free their arms for function by challenging their limits and gaining control of greater amounts of weight shift in all directions.

Biomechanical changes that aid in the development of independent sitting continue to occur. Greater range of hip abduction/external rotation allows the lateral aspect of the leg to have greater surface contact with the floor and provides a larger base of support. As the baby leans forward or diagonally forward over the femur in this position, the hip joint becomes more mobile. This movement component is important for transitions in and out of sitting in later months.

There is a great variety in sitting postures as each baby is unique in regard to postural tone, control of balance, and preferred patterns of postural alignment and movement. Some babies tend to keep their center of gravity more forward over their hips (figure 5.14), although they can briefly sit erect as they recruit more muscle activity of the trunk and pelvic girdle. Some babies are more flexed in the spine and may keep their center of gravity more posterior, tilting the pelvis back slightly. Others sit erect and carefully shift their weight in small ranges over their stable base of support (figure 5.15). They rely less on arm support, but keep their upper arms close to their bodies and often use increased flexion of the elbow and hand for stability.

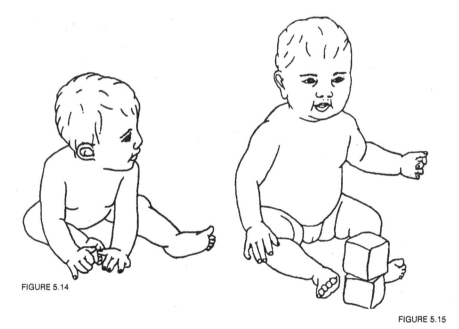

FIGURE 5.14

FIGURE 5.15

A limited variety of lower extremity postures is possible, and the baby may sit with symmetrical flexion of the knees or one knee more extended. Full knee extension is not usually seen at this age because of the amount of external rotation of the hip. The position of the lower extremities is functionally significant. If the knee is more flexed, greater weight shift over the hip is mechanically possible because the hamstrings are allowed to shorten distally (figure 5.16). When the knee is extended, greater stability for upper body activities is achieved. Examples include holding a toy or lifting and turning the head (thoracic rotation) (figure 5.17).

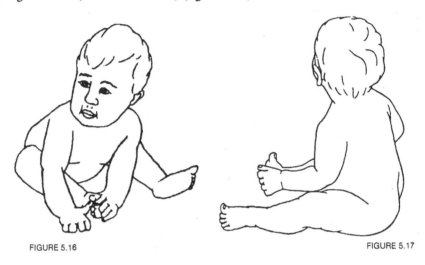

FIGURE 5.16   FIGURE 5.17

Postural synergies that are active in maintaining the sitting position include the erector spinae, abdominals, hip extensors, and sometimes hip flexors. Each baby develops a preferred pattern for holding a posture, controlling weight shift while moving, and returning to that posture. Through motor learning the baby develops coordination of postural control with movement so that sitting is efficient and functional. For example, while leaning forward and returning to the erect position, the baby initially uses the pattern of scapular adduction and thoracic extension to aid in shifting the center of gravity up and back (figure 5.18). As motor learning occurs, the baby uses fewer muscles and joints of the upper body and relies on greater hip activity against the surface with spinal extension from the sacral area upward.

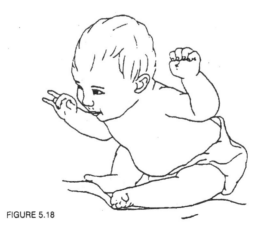

FIGURE 5.18

Six-month-old babies are the most stable when reaching forward and down to the surface. Often they prefer a large toy that gives them more distal stability, and one arm may be used for weight bearing (figure 5.19). Instead of arm support, they may use retraction of the shoulder or humeral extension of one arm to control the center of gravity as they reach with the other. They also easily reach diagonally forward and down to play with their toes and feet. They may attempt a more lateral weight shift, but are more likely to lose their balance or collapse forward. By the end of the sixth month they often begin to rotate to one side and, with bilateral arm support, begin to prepare for transitioning out of sitting to prone.

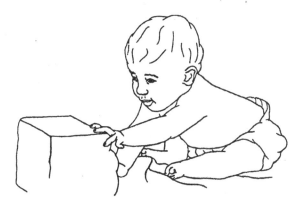

FIGURE 5.19

Standing. The six-month-old child demonstrates greater muscle activity of the abdominals and hip extensors in standing and a narrower base of support is possible (figure 5.20). Rather than abducted, the legs are now vertical to the pelvis and the hips are more extended. Less support is required and the baby may hold on by grasping an adult's fingers rather than being held by the hands or arms. The baby can repetitively flex and extend the hips and knees, pushing with the feet against the floor. This bouncing activity increases strength of lower extremity musculature as well as providing sensory information to the motor control system. Some babies pull to standing in their cribs or take steps with their hands held, but most babies begin these activities in the seventh month.

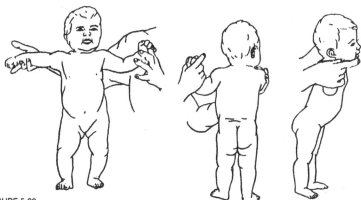

FIGURE 5.20

■ Fine Motor Development

Upper Extremity Development

The six-month-old child is developing more control of the whole body in motion. As the trunk develops, the baby experiences greater control of eyes, arms, and hands. The surrounding world becomes potentially accessible as the baby begins to take risks and reach further into the environment with a sense of curiosity and joy. The baby's mind is collecting data from all sensory systems and, through movements, the baby begins to draw conclusions about the surrounding spatial world.

Prone. In prone, the six-month-old child continues to reach forward, lengthening scapulohumeral and scapulothoracic musculature (figure 5.21). The baby can correct the center of gravity in prone, an indication of greater lateral trunk control (figure 5.22). The baby easily transfers weight to one arm and reaches with dissociation of one side of the body from the other (figure 5.23). The baby does not need to adduct the weight bearing arm against the trunk for stability, as was necessary at five months of age. Instead, the baby pushes the arm against the supporting surface with shoulder girdle depression and is able to maintain that postural control briefly while playing. This visually directed reach strengthens the muscles of the weight-bearing shoulder and hip and encourages development of oblique abdominal activity. Rotation of the upper body over a stable pelvis occurs. This will be utilized in later months as rotation with extension in sitting.

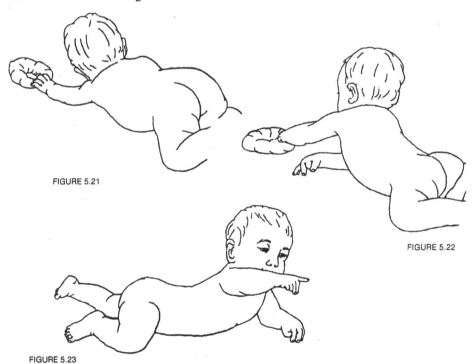

FIGURE 5.21

FIGURE 5.22

FIGURE 5.23

While weight bearing on one arm and reaching with the other, the baby develops isolated control of one shoulder girdle from the other. This is in preparation for the emergence of a unilateral reaching pattern in other positions (figure 5.24). It also prepares the baby for the development of protective responses in sitting.

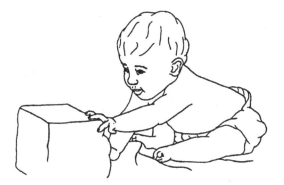

FIGURE 5.24

Due to improved control of vision and auditory localization, the six-month-old baby has a strong desire to move away from the floor. The baby adducts the arms (figure 5.25) and begins to push the weight posteriorly as the hips are flexed (figure 5.26). Although most six-month-old children remain in weight bearing on forearms (figure 5.27), occasionally, the baby may push up asymmetrically on extended arms, using a wide base of upper extremity support and stabilization from the hip flexors (figure 5.28). The baby then briefly scans the environment from a new perspective.

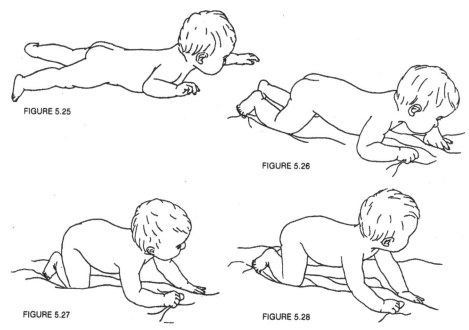

FIGURE 5.25

FIGURE 5.26

FIGURE 5.27

FIGURE 5.28

Sitting. The six-month-old baby has developed protective forward extension and uses this response to support the body while reaching for a toy beyond arms' length (figure 5.29). The baby may utilize the strong scapular adductors to transfer weight toward the hips to regain an upright posture against gravity (figure 5.30).

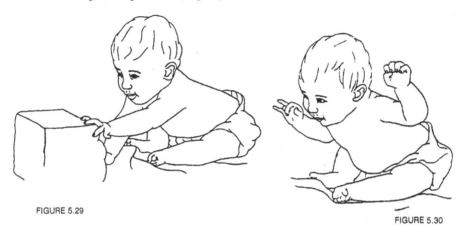

FIGURE 5.29

FIGURE 5.30

With external support from an adult or high chair, the baby can accurately direct the reach forward with full elbow extension. Reach continues to be strongly bilateral due to insufficient lateral trunk control in sitting (figure 5.31). During visual exploration or while moving and shaking a toy, the baby tends to maintain the object close to the body (figure 5.32). As hip activity against the supporting surface is developed, the baby will be able to move the arms freely in space. In other words, freedom of arm function in space is dependent on dynamic pelvic stability.

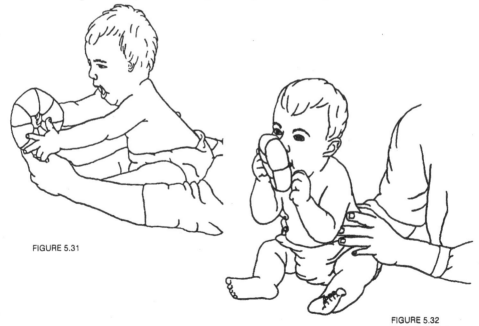

FIGURE 5.31

FIGURE 5.32

Hand Development

Fine motor control in the six-month-old varies with the degree of proximal stability that is provided. For example, in sitting, the baby's range of reach and control of grasp is better when the trunk is supported by an adult than it is when the baby attempts to use the upper extremities in independent sitting. In supine, where the whole spine is stabilized by the supporting surface, the child has optimum control of the whole upper extremity (figure 5.33).

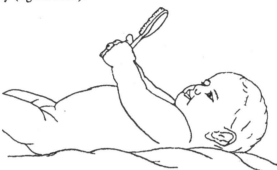

FIGURE 5.33

The baby uses shoulder and elbow motion to move toys through space. The baby shakes and bangs a toy to produce an interesting sound and maintains the grasp of toys that fit well into the palm and explores them through the visual, auditory, and oral systems. Toys that are larger than the palmar arch are more difficult for the baby to maintain because his palmar stability and digital control are not yet fully developed (figure 5.34). The stability in the hand is dependent on the degree of control of the long finger flexors and extensors (Boehme 1988). These long muscle groups originate at the distal end of the humerus, cross over the elbow joint, wrist joint and carpals, and insert into the metacarpals (figure 5.35). With each minute movement in the hand, muscular activity can be palpated in the forearm. As the long finger flexors and extensors develop equal control, the child gains more neutral alignment in the wrist. In general this develops near the end of the sixth month.

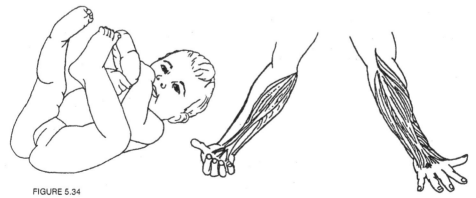

FIGURE 5.34

FIGURE 5.35

The specific patterns of grasp observed at this age are dependent on the size, shape, and firmness of the object held. For example, the baby continues to use a palmar grasp on small dowel-shaped objects. In this case, the object is held with fingers flexed and thumb adducted (Erhardt 1982). The distal digit of the thumb is often flexed (figure 5.36). However, larger objects that fit easily into the palm are held with a radial-palmar grasp (figure 5.37). Here the fingers press the object against the radial side of the hand and opposed thumb (Erhardt 1982). The object itself helps shape the palm and digits. It is through the child's experience with different sizes and shapes that the hand learns new motor accommodations.

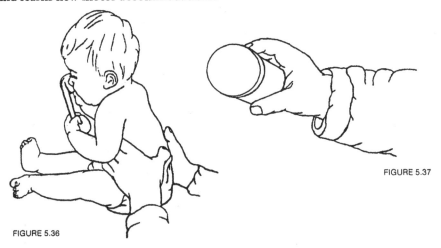

FIGURE 5.37

FIGURE 5.36

The six-month-old child can release an object through a smooth two-stage transfer (figures 5.38, 5.39, and 5.40). The baby uses concentration and effort to accomplish hand-to-hand transfer at this age. The child cannot yet voluntarily release an object in space. Consequently, the baby may fling the object or use a whole arm abduction movement to open the hand for release.

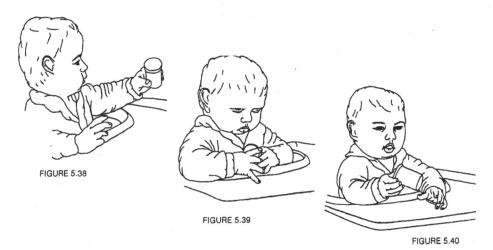

FIGURE 5.38

FIGURE 5.39

FIGURE 5.40

Most six-month-old children are not successful when trying to grasp a pellet-sized object because they have not yet developed isolated control of the fingers. The baby may attempt to trap a tiny object between two fingers or rake the object into the palm. The thumb is adducted into the palm, providing proximal palmar stability as a base for emerging distal digital mobility. The baby gains control of the digits through intrinsic muscle activity between seven and nine months of age.

Functionally, the six-month-old child is already motivated toward self-care. From the babies' perspective, they would rather do it themselves. Often the baby's hands have to be held out of the way during spoon feeding, because the baby tends to pull the spoon out rather than put it in the mouth (figure 5.41). The baby assists with cupdrinking by placing the hands on top of the adult hand (figure 5.42). Although awkward, the child is successful at finger feeding with breadsticks or teething biscuits because of their shape and firmness (figure 5.43). This hand-to-mouth pattern is accomplished with elbow and forearm motion because the baby has not yet developed dynamic movement in the wrist. Babies are usually unsuccessful with crackers as they cannot yet grade the firmness of their hand pressure.

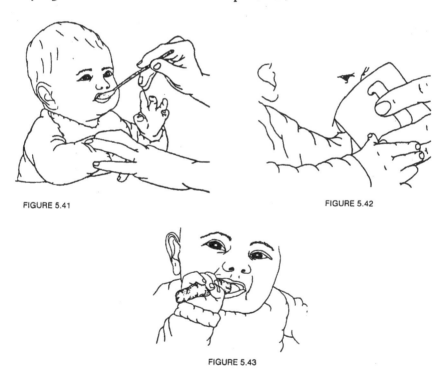

FIGURE 5.41

FIGURE 5.42

FIGURE 5.43

Visual Development

Six-month-old babies have developed the ability to posturally respond to changes in their center of gravity. This allows them to adjust their position in space as they visually locate objects in the environment. Because of greater stability in the cervical spine, the baby also has independent movement of head on neck as demonstrated by the emergence of the anterior, posterior, and lateral labyrinthine and optical righting responses. This, in turn, allows the baby to move the eyes independently from the head. The baby can visually track an object laterally or peripherally through the full oculomotor range (Erhardt 1990).

As the six-month-old develops symmetrical flexion with abdominal oblique activity, consistent binocular fixation and eye convergence can be observed. In addition, as equilibrium reactions develop in prone and begin to emerge in supine, the baby begins to visually track in a diagonal direction. These oculomotor options allow the baby to visually scan several objects in the same or different spatial planes (Erhardt 1990).

Typically, six-month-old babies gain more proximal control, which in turn leads to greater distal control of muscles in the eyes, hands, and mouth. The impact on function is observed in babies' interactions with their world. More consistent interplay is seen between the eyes, hands, and mouth as the babies explore toys visually, tactually, and orally. This multisensory awareness has an important impact on cognitive development. Reach is now visually directed with intention (figures 5.44, 5.45, and 5.46). This conscious, deliberate intent to make contact with and explore a specific object illustrates the six-month-old child's development of object permanence.

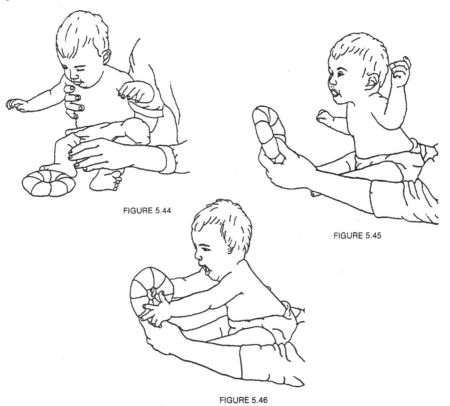

FIGURE 5.44

FIGURE 5.45

FIGURE 5.46

In addition, as the baby develops trunk control in sitting with beginning control of the hips against the supporting surface, attempts may be made to reach beyond arms' length. As the baby's vision projects further into space, the surrounding world expands and the desire to move further in space is strengthened.

Auditory localization parallels development of mobile head control and proximal trunk stability. Localization of sound gives babies more specific information about space in relationship to their physical bodies. The world takes on meaning that directs their actions. Babies begin to understand that there are foreground and background spatial fields and they learn to selectively respond to sounds that are closest, sounds that can be visually and physically explored (Barsch 1968). While conceptualizing the nearby world, babies are motivated to explore and understand that world. Their curiosity is so much stronger than the fear of falling that babies will lunge through space to make contact with the surrounding world.

■ Oral-Motor and Respiratory Development

Anatomical/Structural Characteristics

The oral and pharyngeal mechanisms. As described in Chapter 4, significant modifications in the contour, shape, size, and alignment of the structures and musculature of the oral and pharyngeal mechanisms begin to occur during the period from four to six months of age. Since the eruption of the deciduous teeth is often discussed in regard to the six-month-old child and has a significant influence on the baby's development of new functional activities, it seems appropriate to discuss it more fully at this time.

Twenty deciduous (temporary or primary) teeth are contained within the alveolar processes of the mandible and the maxilla, five on each side (Netter 1959; Hiatt and Gartner 1982). Within each quadrant is a central incisor, lateral incisor, canine (cuspid), first molar, and second molar (figure 5.47).

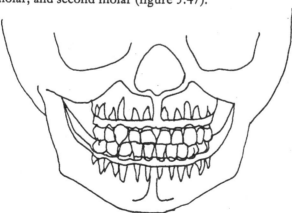

FIGURE 5.47
Adapted from Sicher and DuBrul 1975 (figure 5.62).

Teeth are primarily composed of hard tissue, which, in the deciduous teeth, begins to be formed *in utero*. Each tooth is composed of the part that can be seen in the oral cavity as well as a part that is contained within the alveolus, covering the root (Sicher and DuBrul 1975).

Several factors appear to influence the actual eruption of the deciduous teeth through the dense gingival (gum) tissue, including growth and movements of the tooth within the alveolar processes of the mandible and maxilla, development and growth of the root of the tooth, pressures from the connective tissue and ligaments, and pressures from changes in the skeletal or bony framework the tooth is held in (Sicher and DuBrul 1975). Eruption of the teeth must be viewed as a gradual process that continues over time and not just in terms of the initial breaking through of a tooth into the oral cavity.

There is considerable variation in the development of teeth among individuals (Sicher and DuBrul 1975). Generally, the central incisors of the mandible appear first at approximately six months of age. By approximately nine to ten months of age, the lateral incisors of the mandible as well as the central and lateral incisors of the maxilla have begun to erupt. The first molars of the mandible and maxilla emerge at about 12 to 14 months of age. By 24 to 30 months of age, the mandibular and maxillary canines, or cuspids, and the mandibular and maxillary second molars have erupted, completing the child's primary dentition. The permanent teeth will begin to appear at approximately six years of age often with the emergence of the permanent first molars and then the central and lateral incisors (Ranly 1980).

Rib cage and diaphragm. Changes in the shape and contour of the rib cage initially seen at about four to five months of age are now more consistently evident. Increasing use of the abdominal musculature in prone, supine, sitting, sidelying, and rolling provides input that pulls and rotates the ribs downward. Longer periods spent in sitting and standing allow gravity to influence the contour of the rib cage, pulling it downward. Greater postural activity against gravity and greater abdominal musculature activity assist in changing the shape of the rib cage while elongating the chest wall (Massery 1991).

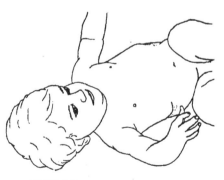

FIGURE 5.48

More experience with controlled shoulder girdle and upper extremity activities also has a dramatic affect on rib cage contour. As the six-month-old child uses musculature of the shoulder girdle and upper extremities in reaching and weight bearing, the upper chest opens up. The upper anterior rib cage appears flatter and less constricted, taking on a more rectangular shape (figure 5.48). This more expanded upper chest area provides greater space in which the upper ribs and sternum can begin to move on inhalation in the near future.

The abdominal muscles are beginning to provide greater stability to the lower rib cage. However, the abdominal obliques are active only intermittently during general movement. They have not yet provided input to the rib cage sufficient to elongate the musculature and soft tissue connecting rib to rib and to prepare the intercostals for active rib cage expansion on inhalation. Therefore, belly-breathing with rib flaring or lower rib expansion on inhalation continues to be evident at six months of age.

Although belly breathing continues to be predominant, modifications in the belly-breathing pattern are present. As the ribs begin to rotate downward, the lumbar spine becomes more active in movement, greater pelvic and hip mobility and stability develop, the trunk elongates and develops greater postural control against gravity, and the diaphragm begins to modify in its shape and movement. The diaphragm becomes more dome-shaped as its lateral, anterior, and posterior muscle fibers lengthen and move downward in conjunction with the downward rotation of the ribs (Massery 1991). There is now more space within the trunk for the diaphragm to move. This results in greater active belly expansion on inhalation, increased air intake, and a reduced respiratory rate in the six-month-old child (figure 5.49).

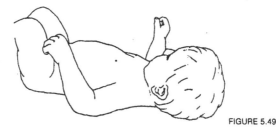

FIGURE 5.49

Developmental Characteristics

The face of a six-month-old child reveals feelings and needs that were once exhibited only through crying or not crying, fussing, and cooing. The baby can now use the facial musculature to produce changes in facial expression. Facial expression, often used in conjunction with eye contact and upper extremity movements (for example, reaching) provides the adult with a more effective means to interpret the infant's likes, dislikes, wants, and needs (figure 5.50).

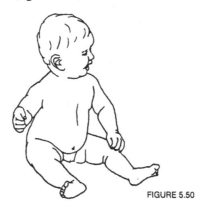

FIGURE 5.50

The use of the oral mechanism continues to be important in exploration and investigation of the environment even as vision and use of the hands are becoming more functional. Six-month-old children often appear to be putting everything they come in contact with into their mouths. This most probably occurs due to a combination of factors that includes the start of teething.

Instead of just suckling or sucking on objects brought into the mouth, the baby now begins to "bite" on objects using small, phasic up and down jaw movements (figure 5.51). Since the cheeks and lips are not active in this process, a great amount of drooling occurs. Direct input into the gums appears to help the baby deal with some of the discomfort caused by swelling of the gums and the slow gradual eruption of teeth through the gum tissue. Through these new oral sensory activities, the six-month-old child discovers new movements of the mouth; experiences more coordinated mouth movements; learns to coordinate mouth movements with breathing, swallowing, upper extremity function, and other body movements; and becomes more aware of how to use the mouth to investigate new toys and objects in the environment.

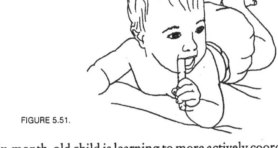

FIGURE 5.51.

The six-month-old child is learning to more actively coordinate oral and pharyngeal function with general movement as greater antigravity motor control and improved postural activity are developed. Longer periods of active lip closure are maintained in supine (figure 5.52), prone (figure 5.53), and sitting (figure 5.54). In prone and

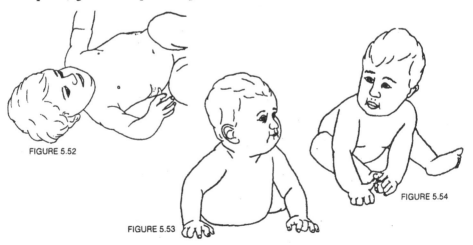

FIGURE 5.52

FIGURE 5.53

FIGURE 5.54

sitting, greater postural control provides a foundation from which the baby is freer to experience a greater variety of active lip, jaw, and tongue movements (figures 5.55, 5.56, 5.57, and 5.58) with less need to use the oral mechanism positionally to provide and reinforce stability. In newer activities, such as standing, sidelying, and rolling, the six-month-old child may exhibit greater positional use of the oral mechanism for stability and less variety of active oral movements (figures 5.59 and 5.60).

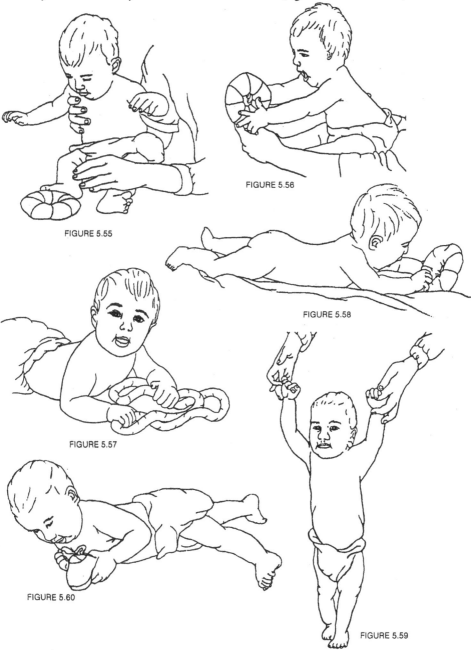

FIGURE 5.55

FIGURE 5.56

FIGURE 5.57

FIGURE 5.58

FIGURE 5.59

FIGURE 5.60

The feeding process. The oral-motor function of six-month-old children during feeding and drinking tasks reflects the experience they have gained in learning to coordinate oral movements and new oral and pharyngeal structural alignment with greater active postural control against gravity. In addition, they exhibit a readiness to experience new oral movements, new food textures, new feeding activities, and new feeding positions.

The six-month-old child continues to be held in a semi-reclined position by the adult for bottledrinking or breastfeeding. The baby may continue to be fed semisolids by spoon while sitting in an infant seat or car seat, often requiring less of an angle of recline than was needed at four to five months of age. Many six-month-old babies are also being introduced to feeding and cupdrinking while in a highchair because their postural activity in sitting is now more controlled, allowing them to be at a 90-degree angle. Some adaptations in the highchair are often required to limit their potential of falling laterally and to allow them to focus on feeding without having to work hard to maintain an upright posture. A more secure upright position in the highchair allows the baby to coordinate the oral, pharyngeal, and respiratory mechanisms more effectively and efficiently for feeding.

Sucking is the predominant oral-motor pattern used by the six-month-old baby during bottledrinking and breastfeeding (figure 5.61). The lips actively surround and hold on to the nipple so that no liquid loss occurs during the sucking process. The cheek musculature draws inward providing a foundation of active stability for the lips and oral cavity, which assists in creating the intra-oral negative pressure characteristic of sucking. The tongue cups, surrounds, and strongly holds on to the nipple within the oral cavity as it moves in an up/down direction, making it extremely difficult for the feeder to remove the nipple from the mouth while the infant is actively sucking. The jaw moves in smaller, more graded up/down movements while the nipple is in the mouth. The six-month-old baby produces long sequences of coordinated sucking, swallowing, and breathing during bottledrinking and breastfeeding.

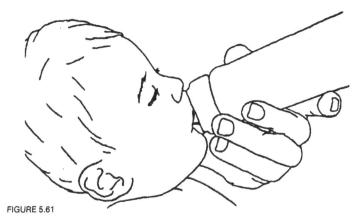

FIGURE 5.61

Movements of the oral mechanism characteristic of suckling are still used by the infant. They are seen most often when the nipple is initially brought to the mouth, when the nipple is removed from the mouth, and when the infant starts or stops the sucking process. Liquid loss may occur whenever suckling is being used.

The six-month-old child is becoming a more active participant in bottledrinking and breastfeeding. The baby visually recognizes the bottle or breast, opens the mouth, and holds the mouth open with a quiet tongue and jaw as the nipple is brought toward and into the mouth. The baby may try to assist by bringing the hands up to hold the bottle. The automatic phasic bite-release pattern and rooting response no longer influence the baby's activities because voluntary control of head, neck, and oral movements has emerged.

Although bottledrinking and breastfeeding will continue to be the primary sources for liquid intake, cupdrinking is often introduced by six months of age. Movements of the oral mechanism characteristic of suckling predominate as the baby begins to experience this new, more advanced task. The tongue moves rhythmically forward and backward as the jaw moves primarily in wide up/down excursions with minimal lip closure. Liquid loss occurs. Problems in coordinating sequences of suckling, swallowing, and breathing and in successfully controlling the amount of liquid entering the mouth may result in coughing and choking.

When the adult places and holds the cup firmly in the mouth, the baby may modify the oral-motor activity (figure 5.62). The lower lip moves up and out, stabilizing against the cup. This stability provided through the cup placement by the feeder and by the baby's lower lip allows for experience with brief periods of more organized and coordinated tongue, jaw, and lip activity like that used for sucking. When the cup is removed or reinserted, suckling is again noted as the baby attempts to reorganize oral movements on a less stable base.

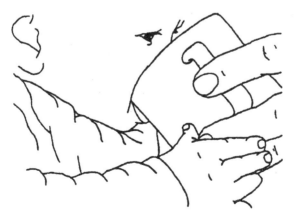

FIGURE 5.62

When not involved in another activity while in the highchair, the six-month-old child shows visual recognition of the spoon, opening the mouth and keeping the tongue and jaw quiet as the spoon approaches (figure 5.63). As the spoon enters the mouth, the jaw elevates, the lower lip moves up and out to stabilize under the spoon, and the upper lip moves down toward the food. This downward movement of the upper lip allows the feeder to bring the spoon out on a more horizontal plane so food can be scraped off on the downwardly-postured upper lip (figure 5.64).

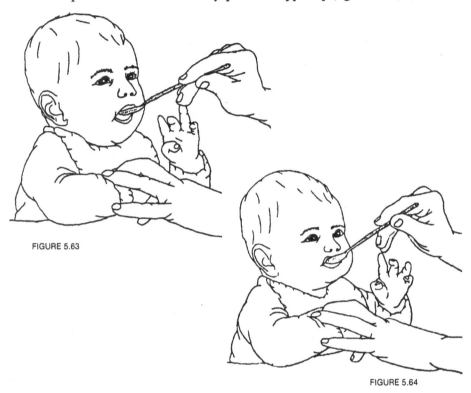

FIGURE 5.63

FIGURE 5.64

Smooth, pureed food is moved back in the oral mechanism for swallowing, using predominantly suckling with some sucking movements of the tongue, jaw, and lips. The tongue protrudes between the lips as the final remnants of food are cleared from the oropharyngeal area. If the child has had previous experience with the semisolid texture presented, gagging generally does not occur. As the cheeks and lips become more active and tongue and jaw movements become more coordinated and refined, less food will be lost from the mouth during spoonfeeding.

Hard solids and soft solids placed in the front of the mouth are handled in much the same manner as discussed in Chapter 4 for the five-month-old child. Small phasic up/ down movements of the jaw, sucking, or suckling are produced when the solid is placed in the front of the mouth. The six-month-old child may begin to exhibit a more variable up/down motion of the jaw with flattening and up/down motions of the tongue, which is characteristic of the earliest chewing pattern called munching

(Morris and Klein 1987). If pieces accidentally break off and do not adequately mix with saliva, the baby either spits them out or swallows them whole. Gagging or choking occurs if a piece falls to the back of the tongue.

If a solid is placed on the side of the mouth between the biting surfaces of the gums, the six-month-old baby begins to use new oral activity in response (figures 5.65 and 5.66). When food is placed and held on the side biting surfaces, the baby's tongue moves to that side. As the tongue moves laterally, the movements of the jaw begin to change. Opening and closing of the jaw now begins to include lateral and downward movements in conjunction with lateral tongue activity. Because of the musculature and structural alignment of the jaw, these lateral and downward jaw movements appear to be in a diagonal plane of movement. Some asymmetrical tightening of the cheek and lip musculature on the side where the food is placed may also be evident. Once a piece of solid comes off and moves to the center of the tongue, suckling or sucking results.

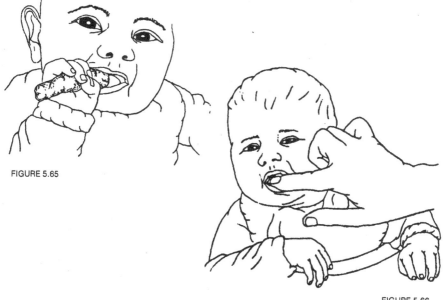

FIGURE 5.65

FIGURE 5.66

Significant components of respiratory function. Belly breathing continues to be the infant's predominant respiratory pattern. However, changes in the angle and contour of the rib cage and the alignment and shape of the diaphragm now result in deeper inhalation evidenced by greater belly expansion. Increased air intake provides greater air flow available for sound production during exhalation. Therefore, the six-month-old child produces sounds that are longer in duration.

As the ribs move downward and the abdominal musculature becomes more active, the shoulder girdle depresses and becomes a more stable foundation for the oral and pharyngeal mechanisms. This allows the child to more easily coordinate oral, pharyngeal, and respiratory function during general movement, feeding, swallowing, and sound production activities. Changes in the shape and alignment of the structures of the pharyngeal area result in a greater variety of intonation and pitch changes during longer phonation.

Sounds continue to be generated with active body movements. As the alignment of the tongue within the oral and pharyngeal mechanisms modifies and the extrinsic tongue musculature provides a more active point of stability for tongue body movements, the six-month-old baby begins to make sounds that are specifically produced with the front or back of the tongue (figure 5.67). Initially these new consonant sounds are produced during feeding and other oral sensory activities.

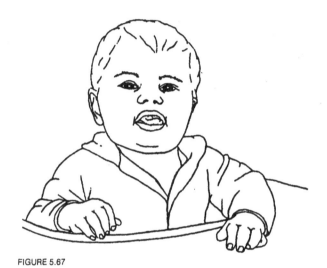

FIGURE 5.67

Eruption of the teeth may result in new sounds being produced. As the baby brings the tongue or lips in contact with newly emerging central incisors on exhalation, new sounds using tongue-to-teeth or lip-to-teeth contact are produced.

Summary Chart—6 Months

Postural Control	Gross Motor	Reach	Fine Motor	Vision
Trunk righting reaction present when tipped in space	*Supine* • holds arms and legs vertical • rolls to side and prone	In prone, can weight shift and reach with control	Consistent palmar grasp	Fully developed visual control
Landau reaction mature	Uses sidelying as a position for play; may weightbear on one foot	Continues to primarily use bilateral reach in sitting, supine, and sidelying	Radial-palmar grasp emerging	Eye movements independent from head movements
Forward protective extension of the arms	*Prone* • stretches arms forward • plays with a variety of forearm and extended arm positions		Transfers hand to hand	
Equilibrium reactions in prone and supine	• trunk elongation and lower extremity extension pattern on one side with trunk lateral flexion and lower extremity on the other side	Unilateral reach emerging as pelvic and hip control develop	Attempts to help with spoonfeeding and cupdrinking	
Body-on-body righting response with spinal rotation	• begins to assume quadruped • tries to move self on floor		Fingerfeeds with bread sticks or teething biscuits	
Increased postural activity of lower body for maintaining postures and to accompany volitional movements	Rolls between supine, sidelying, and prone with control; able to stop at various points or to roll consecutively	Consistent visually directed reach	Shakes and bangs toys to create auditory and visual effect	
	Sitting • sits well in high chair; enjoys bounce-type seats • begins to sit independently with arm support			
Lateral weight shift through lower trunk and pelvis in prone	• may reach with one arm while supporting with other • may sit briefly with no arm support but falls easily			
Greater control for unilateral movements and asymmetrical postures	*Standing* • feet closer together • greater hip extension • requires less support • bounces			

Some infants develop activities earlier or later than this chart indicates. Therefore, it should not be regarded as a rigid timetable of events.

Summary Chart–6 Months continued

Oral-Motor/Feeding	Respiration-Phonation
Rooting response and automatic phasic bite-release pattern not present	*Respiration* Belly breathing with greater belly expansion on inhalation
Gag response diminishing in strength	Coordinates breathing more easily with general movement, feeding, swallowing, and sound production
Feeding Sucks liquid from bottle/breast with no liquid loss and long sequences of coordinated sucking-swallowing-breathing; suckles on nipple insertion/removal	*Phonation/Sounds* Vocalizes pleasure/displeasure
Suckles liquid presented by cup • may bring lower lip up under cup held in mouth • loses liquid • coughs/chokes when takes in too much liquid and with uncoordinated suckling-swallowing-breathing	Babbles longer repetitive sound sequences with greater loudness, pitch, and intonation variations
	In sitting, produces sounds with greater lip and tongue control/movements
Opens/quiets mouth as spoon approaches • brings lower lip up under spoon • moves upper lip down so food is scraped off on it • uses suckling with some sucking to move food back • may protrude tongue on swallow • some food loss • gags on new semisolid textures	Begins producing consonants with front and back of tongue
Uses phasic up/down jaw movements, suckling, or sucking with solids placed in front • may begin munching • gags/chokes on pieces that fall to back of tongue	If teeth have erupted, produces sounds with lip-to-teeth and tongue-to-teeth contact
Moves tongue laterally with solids placed on side biting surfaces • moves jaw laterally and downward (diagonally) as tongue lateralizes • sucks/suckles pieces on center of tongue	Produces phonation/sounds in direct relationship to body movement
Oral-Motor Uses facial expressions that convey likes/dislikes	
Sucks, suckles, and uses up/down jaw movements to investigate new objects	
Maintains lip closure longer in supine, prone, and sitting	
Produces greater variety of lip, jaw, and tongue movements in prone and sitting	
May posture mouth for stability in standing, sidelying, and rolling	
Drools when babbling, reaching, and teething; drools less during feeding	

■ References

Barsch, R. H. 1968. *Achieving perceptual-motor efficiency*. Seattle, WA: Special Child Publications.

Boehme, R. 1988. *Improving upper body control*. Tucson, AZ: Therapy Skill Builders.

Caplan, F. 1971. *The first twelve months of life*. New York: Grosset and Dunlap.

Erhardt, R. P. 1982. *Developmental hand dysfunction theory assessment treatment*. Tucson, AZ: Therapy Skill Builders.

_____. 1990. *Developmental visual dysfunction models for assessment and management*. Tucson, AZ: Therapy Skill Builders.

Hiatt, J. L., and L. P. Gartner. 1982. *Textbook of head and neck anatomy*. New York: Appleton-Century-Crofts.

Massery, M. 1991. Chest development as a component of normal motor development: Implications for pediatric physical therapists. *Pediatric Physical Therapy* 3(1):3-8.

Morris, S. E., and M. D. Klein. 1987. *Pre-Feeding skills*. Tucson, AZ: Therapy Skill Builders.

Netter, F. H. 1959. Digestive system. In *CIBA collection of medical illustrations*, Vol. 3, edited by E. Oppenheimer, 12-13. Summit, NJ: CIBA Pharmaceutical.

Ranly, D. M. 1980. *A synopsis of craniofacial growth*. New York: Appleton-Century-Crofts.

Sicher, H., and E. L. DuBrul. 1975. *Oral anatomy*. St. Louis, MO: C. V. Mosby.

Chapter 6

7-9 Months

■ Postural Control

After the sixth month, babies spend little time in prone or supine; rather they sit, get up on their hands and knees, and pull to stand. Considerable postural stability is required to maintain these more upright positions. In particular, pelvic/hip stability increases from seven to nine months and is coordinated with head, shoulder girdle, and trunk control in a variety of positions. In sitting, the baby now pushes the ischial tuberosities against the supporting surface, activating postural musculature, which elongates the trunk and stabilizes the upper body. The ischial tuberosities are the posterior portions of the base of the pelvis that serve as the weight-bearing surface in sitting. This activity is extremely important for free movement of the arms in a sitting position (figure 6.1). In addition to pushing on the hand or forearm in sidelying, the baby also uses the hip against the surface to activate the trunk and

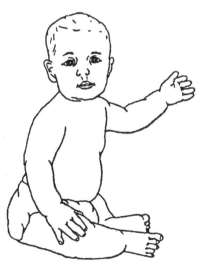

FIGURE 6.1

shoulder girdle. Synergistic activity of all proximal areas is crucial for function in quadruped and for transitioning from one position to another. The baby activates more postural tone when stability is needed (to accompany movement). At other times, the baby relaxes the postural musculature and tends to hang on the structural support provided by the skeleton and soft tissue (figure 6.2).

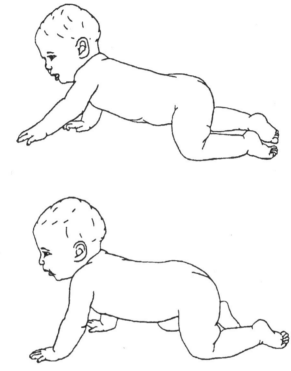

FIGURE 6.2

The seven- to nine-month-old child is capable of many functional motor skills and uses movement to interact with the environment. Postural activity must provide stability and control weight shifts during these movements. Postural accompaniments to focal movement patterns develop as part of motor learning. For example, in sitting, the baby learns to control displacement of the center of gravity while rotating the trunk in order to reach. Locomotion is possible in quadruped because body weight can be shifted from one set of supporting limbs to another. The baby can get into standing by pulling the center of gravity up with the arms, moving the legs under the body, and shifting the weight up and back over the pelvis. The baby also begins to develop postural activity for functional movement in standing while learning to play and take steps along furniture.

In addition to modulating postural activity during the performance of a motor skill, the baby learns to adapt the posture prior to a movement. The baby may change posture so that it is mechanically more efficient to move over the base of support. For example, in sitting, the baby tucks one leg in toward the pelvis to let the center of gravity move smoothly over the hip in transitioning to that side (figure 6.3). Another way to prepare for a movement is to widen the base of support for increased stability. In quadruped, the baby learns to move one knee forward when reaching in a wide range (figure 6.4). When standing at furniture, the baby steps sideways with one leg to spread the feet further apart prior to reaching for a toy.

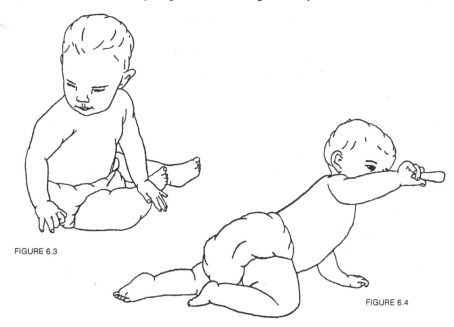

FIGURE 6.3

FIGURE 6.4

Another set of strategies to maintain posture consists of the feedback-based postural reactions that continue to develop during these months. Equilibrium reactions are consistent in prone and supine by seven months. By eight months they are present in sitting and beginning in quadruped. Also, protective extension of the arm is present when the baby's center of gravity is moved sideways or diagonally back to one side (figure 6.5).

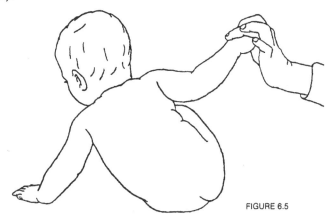

FIGURE 6.5

Postural reactions occur when balance is challenged by an outside force or when babies lose control of their center of gravity during a movement. The latter is seen frequently during this stage of development as babies learn to control postural activity with movement. For example, babies may lose their balance when the head moves backward as they bring an object to the mouth. They are able to regain control by flexing the trunk, abducting the hips, and extending the knees (figure 6.6).

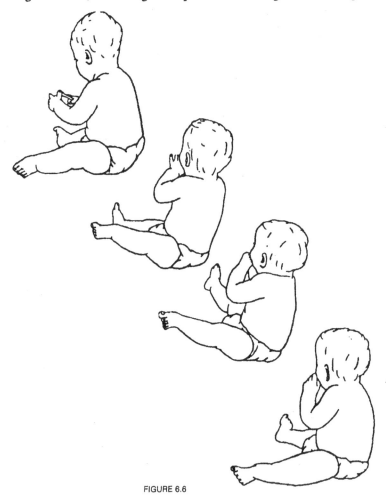

FIGURE 6.6

■ Gross Motor Development

Motor activity surges during this stage and the child develops the skills necessary to explore the expanding environment. The seven- to nine-month-old child rarely stays in supine; in prone the baby is busy reaching, weight shifting, and trying to move along the floor. The spine rotates in a larger excursion, postural activity stabilizes the pelvis and hips, and the lower extremities assume patterns that provide a more dynamic base of support for the upper body (figure 6.7). Thus, the baby can more efficiently orientate body position to desired activities or objects in the environment through a variety of postures.

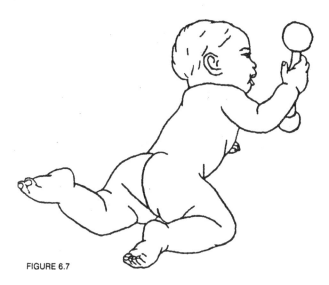

FIGURE 6.7

Rolling to the side, the baby pushes up on one arm to a position in which a large area can be visually and manually explored (figure 6.8). This requires lateral mobility of the trunk, including spinal and rib cage motion as well as soft tissue extensibility. The hip bears most of the weight and the upper leg is free to move into a variety of patterns. Often the foot is active against the floor, providing distal stability. As balance and coordination improve, the child raises the trunk higher off the surface

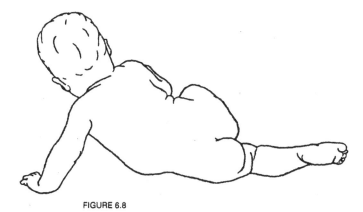

FIGURE 6.8

until close to a sitting position. This is a very dynamic position and a variety of patterns are used as the child reaches in different directions or transitions to other positions (figure 6.9). By eight months, the child can move easily from here to quadruped.

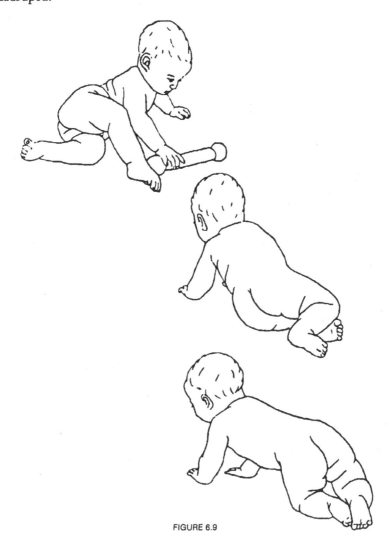

FIGURE 6.9

Sitting. By seven months of age, many babies begin to sit independently with their arms free for play. However, some may still prefer to support themselves on one hand as they reach. As previously stated, each child develops balance and postural control at an individual rate and in an individual pattern. Babies learn to maintain a more erect trunk for longer periods. In addition to erector spinae and abdominal activity, hip extensor musculature must provide postural stability to the base of the pelvis for this to occur. When pelvic stability and control of weight shift is adequate, the baby gives up the arm support except when transitioning to another position. This frees the hands for reach and play so that, from seven to nine months of age, the baby progressively moves the arms in a greater range up and away from the body (figure 6.10).

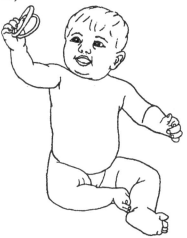

FIGURE 6.10

Sitting becomes more dynamic as the baby is able to shift the weight in wider ranges without falling and in triplanar motions as well as straight planes (figure 6.11). From seven to nine months of age, the baby responds to the environment with more trunk rotation, and the postural accompaniments to the movement include the appropriate amounts of flexion, extension, lateral flexion, and hip/lower extremity activity.

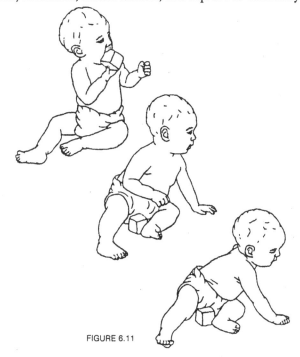

FIGURE 6.11

As stability and postural control increase, the baby develops a greater variety of sitting postures. By eight months of age, the baby often sits with the lower portion of one leg closer to the body (figure 6.12). The key components of this position are the extreme hip external rotation and knee flexion. The amount of hip flexion and abduction vary depending on the activity. The biomechanics of this position require more postural control as it diminishes and changes the shape of the base of support. However, ultimately this position is more functional than the symmetrical ring sitting posture for reaching, playing, and transitioning to other positions.

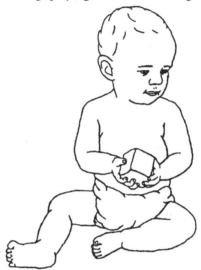

FIGURE 6.12

A variety of lower-extremity postures is crucial for efficient upper extremity function. A baby sits and plays with an object only briefly, then drops or throws it and reaches again. Moving the trunk over the hips and legs, the baby learns to efficiently reach in the surrounding space. The lower extremities assume postures that provide dynamic and mechanical stability for movement of the upper body. In reaching diagonally forward, the baby brings the foot in close while flexing and abducting the opposite hip (figure 6.13). As the baby rotates to reach objects on the floor, the pelvis flexes over

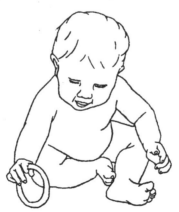

FIGURE 6.13

the femur on the side the baby is reaching to, and the opposite leg biomechanically follows the pelvis so that the knee is facing upward and the foot is weight bearing (figure 6.14). In the nine-month-old child, hip mobility has increased and the hip opposite to the reach internally rotates (figure 6.15). The child now begins to side sit, one hip externally rotated and the other internally rotated.

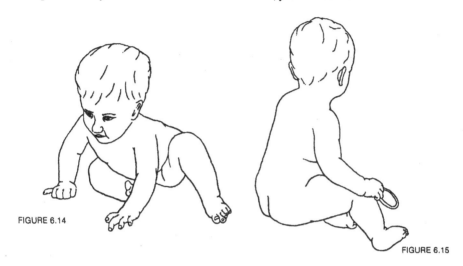

FIGURE 6.14

FIGURE 6.15

Very active babies may bounce in sitting by shifting their body weight forward and back repetitively. The pelvis lifts off the floor as momentum increases, and a forward progression may result. By nine months of age, the baby turns the body ninety degrees or more in sitting. With the leg flexed/abducted/externally rotated, the baby uses the arm to pull the body sideways and pivot over the hip.

Transitions in and out of sitting. By seven months of age, the baby is able to get into a sitting position independently, but only from a quadruped position. Although attempting to sit up from sidelying, the baby is unsuccessful until 10 or 11 months of age and does not sit up symmetrically from supine until five or six years of age. In quadruped, the baby shifts the weight laterally over one knee. The trunk on that side elongates and the opposite side shortens as the pelvis drops. As the buttocks approach the floor, the baby moves the leg forward on the elongated side using hip flexion/abduction/external rotation (figure 6.16). (When this is not done, the baby has to shift the pelvis back over the leg, and the trunk moves too far behind the arms. This is an inefficient pattern because the baby needs to walk the arms backward in order to sit upright.) The baby then can shift the center of gravity to midline and sit erect to free the arms.

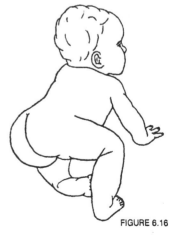

FIGURE 6.16

The seven-month-old child also begins to transition from sitting to prone. With the hip in flexion/abduction/external rotation, the child can move the center of gravity over the pelvis by rotating the trunk. The child places the hands on the floor but cannot sufficiently support the weight shift. Falling forward over the arms, the legs extend behind the body and the baby lands prone on the abdomen. With repetition, the baby learns to assume quadruped by rotating less and increasing knee flexion to control the weight shift while moving the center of gravity diagonally forward onto the arms.

By eight months, the baby develops sufficient shoulder girdle, trunk, and pelvic control to rotate from sitting to quadruped. Now the baby can flex the knee and bring the lower leg closer to the trunk while rotating and leaning to that side. The baby places the hands on the floor, supporting the weight shifting to the arms, and moves the buttocks and unweighted leg into position (figure 6.17). In the next month, coordination and postural control improve so that the movement is performed more easily and quickly.

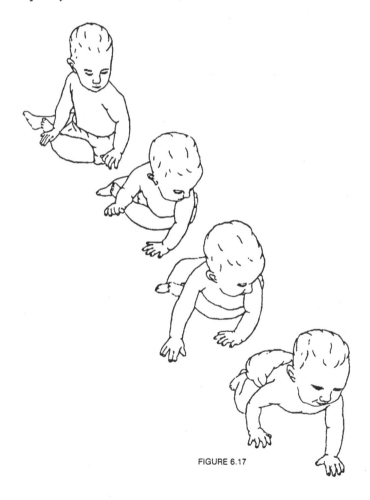

FIGURE 6.17

By nine months of age, babies have increased hip mobility as well as postural control and may use a variety of patterns to move from sitting to quadruped. In addition to rotating over one hip, the baby may tuck in one leg and move directly forward onto the arms (figure 6.18). Full range of external rotation is required as the pelvis moves over the femur and most of the weight is supported on the arms and the tucked leg. The other leg moves into more hip adduction/extension/internal rotation so the knee is in a position for weight bearing. The tucked leg can then internally rotate so the foot is behind the hip.

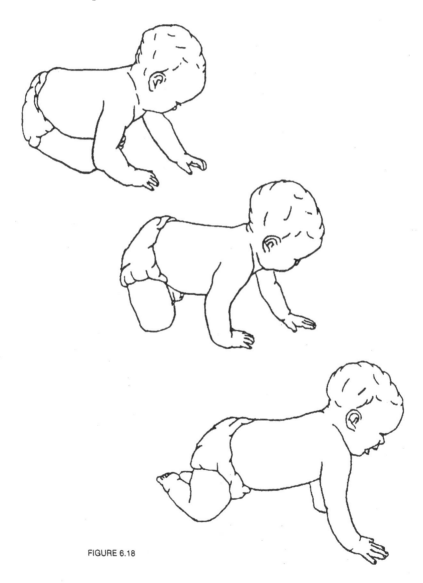

FIGURE 6.18

Another pattern is used to transition from sitting to quadruped (figure 6.19). As the baby reaches diagonally forward over the tucked leg, the opposite foot moves into a position for weight bearing. The baby continues to move the center of gravity forward and the hip extends to place the knee on the floor. The baby may not complete this last step, but rather stay in a hands/knee/foot position to reach for a toy and then lower the body back to sitting.

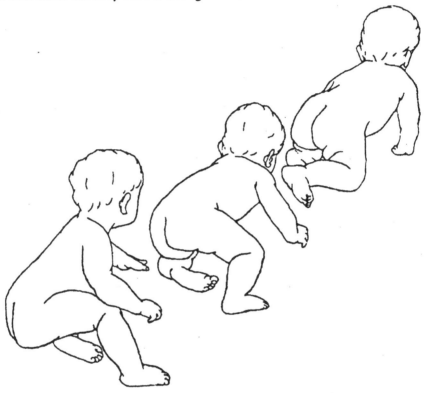

FIGURE 6.19

Quadruped. Pulling the knees up under the abdomen in prone, the seven-month-old baby symmetrically pushes the arms straight to assume the all-fours position. This differs from the six-month-old baby who extended one arm and then the other. The seven-month-old baby now begins to rock forward and back, often losing balance and falling to prone. Postural stability, strength, and coordination develop as the baby shifts the weight, improving shoulder, pelvic, and hip control. Motivated by the vestibular and kinesthetic input, this important activity is performed frequently and prepares for postural control during creeping.

Individual variations of posture are seen in quadruped dependent on the baby's postural activity, joint stability, and motor learning. For example, a baby whose ligaments and joint capsules are more lax may have a sagging belly and lordosis with greater hip flexion. Another may hold the spine straight with little effort. Many babies use shoulder elevation, internal rotation, and finger flexion for upper extremity stability (figure 6.20).

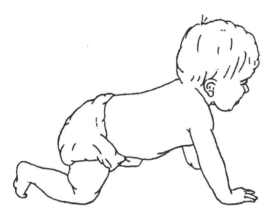

FIGURE 6.20

One important aspect of normal development is the variety of patterns available to accomplish a motor skill. In the eighth and ninth months, babies become proficient in assuming quadruped from different positions using a variety of patterns. In prone, babies learn to simultaneously push on their arms and pull their knees under their hips. They may prefer to symmetrically push up on their arms and bring one leg under the body at a time. The biomechanics of a specific posture favor certain patterns and influence which pattern will be used. A variation of quadruped may occur when one leg is flexed/abducted/externally rotated. The baby can push up on the arms and contract the abdominals, raising the pelvis up to be in a hands-knee-foot position (figure 6.21). Initially, the baby cannot control the hips, but by nine months the baby uses this position for play and creeping. The baby also assumes this position and the hands-and-knees quadruped from sidelying or sitting.

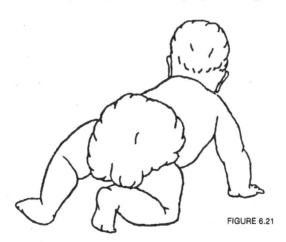

FIGURE 6.21

From seven to nine months of age, the baby learns to control the center of gravity in quadruped and to reach in wider ranges. For example, the baby develops the ability to reach laterally as well as forward (figure 6.22). Initially, symmetrical lower extremity flexion provides stability to support the movement (a). While reaching further and higher, the baby controls the weight shift more efficiently by positioning one knee more forward and the other back, enlarging the base of support (b). In this way, postural activity prepares for the movement and supports the reach. The postural synergies that develop in quadruped become part of the motor program for specific skills, such as pulling to stand at furniture (c).

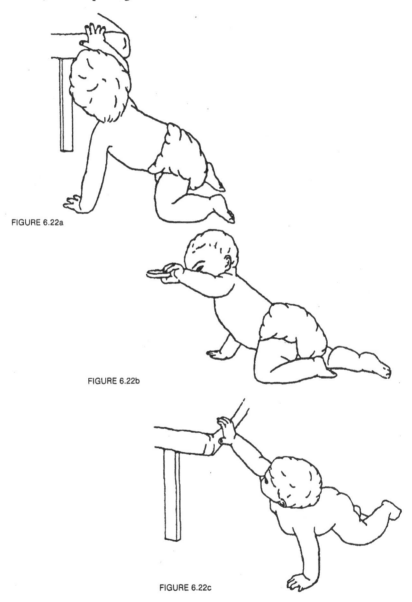

FIGURE 6.22a

FIGURE 6.22b

FIGURE 6.22c

Once mastered, quadruped is a position used to transition to other positions or to locomote. The baby doesn't stay in quadruped, but rather moves into it to get somewhere or something. The baby creeps, looks, reaches, sits and plays, and creeps to another object or pulls to standing. Experimenting with a variety of postures, the baby often stops in the middle of a transition. For example, the baby may lower the pelvis on one side toward a sidelying position, then come back to quadruped (figure 6.23).

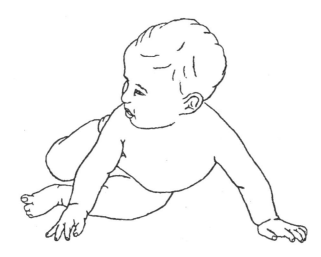

FIGURE 6.23

From prone or quadruped, the baby pushes up on the hands and feet, assuming the plantigrade position (figure 6.24). Appearing to enjoy this movement for its own sake, the baby repeats it many times in succession. This position requires the feet actively pushing against the floor and proximal postural stability, including abdominal activity. Some babies walk their hands and feet forward in a reciprocal pattern.

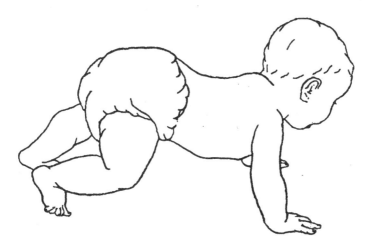

FIGURE 6.24

Locomotion. The seven-month-old baby usually begins to move on the abdomen by pivoting sideways. Leading with the head, shoulders, and upper body, the baby alternately weight shifts from one side to the other. The baby then learns to pull the body forward with the arms in a similar pattern and, although the legs may reciprocate, their action is not propulsive. Initial excursion is small, usually just enough to get a toy that is a little further than the baby's reach. Then the baby begins to pivot or belly crawl in larger ranges and locomotes from one point to another. Many seven-month-old babies move on their abdomens to get where they want to go, while others begin to use four-point creeping as their primary method of locomotion.

Initially, the baby creeps on hands and knees slowly and deliberately. The pattern may not be well coordinated as the baby first moves an arm, then the contralateral leg. Soon the baby begins to move the arm and leg simultaneously. Often the weight-bearing arm does not support the body weight and the baby collapses. With continued practice, motor learning occurs and a smooth pattern emerges.

Early creeping is reciprocal but characterized by lateral flexion/elongation of the trunk as the weight is shifted, simulating the "toddling" of baby's first steps (figure 6.25). Postural control is not yet sufficient to control the movement of the center of gravity. By the ninth month there is less lateral excursion of the trunk and improved hip control. However, diagonal control that requires more rotation is not present until 10 to 11 months of age.

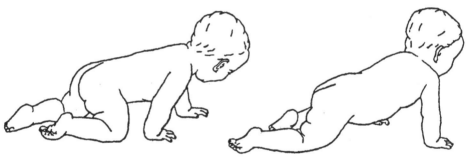

FIGURE 6.25

As with all motor skills, babies vary greatly as to when they begin creeping and how much they use it. While some are proficient by the ninth month, others may not creep readily until they are 10 or 11 months old. A few babies prefer other patterns of locomotion and rarely crawl, although they have the ability to perform the skill. Some babies are content to stay in one room and others creep all over the house, crawling over objects in their path. They may begin to use the same pattern in a vertical direction by climbing up on an adult's lap or up the stairs.

Pulling to stand. Around seven months of age, babies begin to pull themselves to a standing position. The first time may be in the crib and parents are surprised to find their baby standing as they walk into the room. From prone or quadruped, the baby pulls the body up to standing, using the arms to climb the rails. When seated on the floor, an adult's lap is another optimal support for first pulling to standing (figure 6.26). The adult may facilitate the activity by limiting lateral movement of the baby's center of gravity so the baby cannot fall over while moving the legs forward.

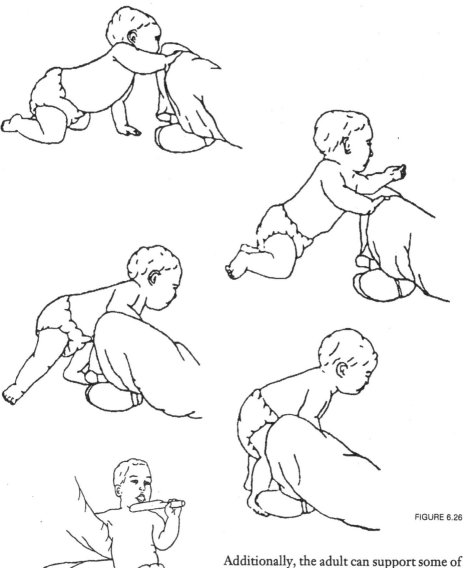

FIGURE 6.26

FIGURE 6.27

Additionally, the adult can support some of the upper body weight so the baby needs less strength to lift the head, shoulders, and trunk to stand upright. Holding on to an adult is a secure way to begin standing, and a baby can lean against the adult's arm and challenge balance by reaching or twisting the trunk (figure 6.27).

When crawling along the floor, the baby tries to pull up on various objects of an optimal size and height, such as footstools, coffee tables, or toy boxes. The baby learns which objects are the most stable and which are not adequate. For example, holding on to a wheeled toy while attempting to stand, the baby discovers that the toy moves. If a surface is too high, the baby cannot shift weight on to the arms and pull. The baby adapts by using a nearby lower surface to get on the hands and feet and then reaching to the higher surface.

The same basic motor pattern is used to pull to standing regardless of the support; however, the baby learns to adapt it for specific situations (figure 6.28). From quadruped, the baby reaches up with one arm, then the other arm, and walks the

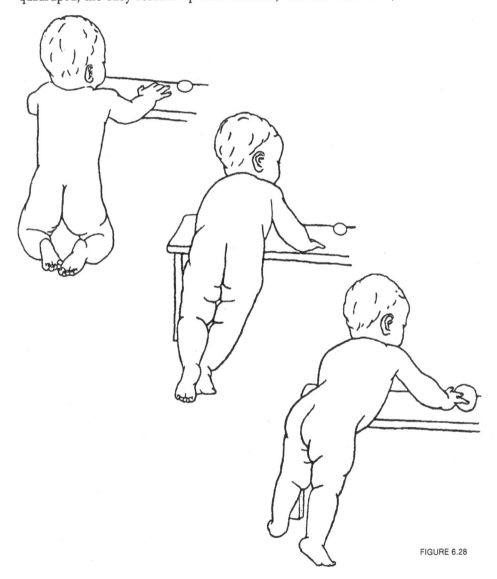

FIGURE 6.28

knees forward. In the first months of standing up, the baby does not assume an upright kneeling position. Rather the knees stay behind the shoulders as postural activity is insufficient to hold the hips extended. Leaning the body forward, the baby pulls with the arms; the pelvis rises and the legs extend symmetrically. Since most of the body weight is on the arms and upper trunk, the baby can walk the legs forward so they are aligned under the pelvis. The baby then pushes on the arms and brings the head, shoulders, and trunk up and back over the hips. A baby in a crib walks the hands up the rails and brings the legs forward.

Around nine or ten months of age, the pattern begins to change as the baby develops more control of the hips. The baby now kneels more upright with the pelvis and hips aligned under the shoulders. Also the weight shifts slightly laterally, elongating that side and shortening the other. Some babies are able to shift far enough to abduct and flex the unweighted hip, bringing the foot forward (figure 6.29). However, they cannot push down on the foot and use the leg to get to standing until later. Rather they continue to shift their weight forward and pull with their arms.

While pulling up, the baby may stop in the kneeling position and reach for a toy. However, there is not sufficient postural control to functionally use the hands in this position. Therefore, the baby lowers the buttocks and sits on the heels to play (figure 6.30).

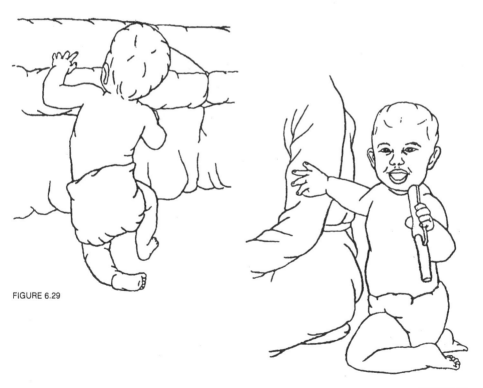

FIGURE 6.29

FIGURE 6.30

Around eight months of age, the baby also pulls to standing from a sitting position. Often this occurs in the crib or playpen, but a low surface such as a footstool may also be used. A baby sitting sideways to the support (figure 6.31) will rotate the upper body and move both arms onto the support. Leaning forward and pushing down with the arms results in the pelvis rising off the floor. Typical of this age, the lower extremities are not active early in the pattern and need to move into a position for weight bearing. If sitting directly in front of the support, the baby uses a similar pattern. Shifting the weight to the arms until the buttocks are unweighted, the baby places the feet on the floor and extends the knees.

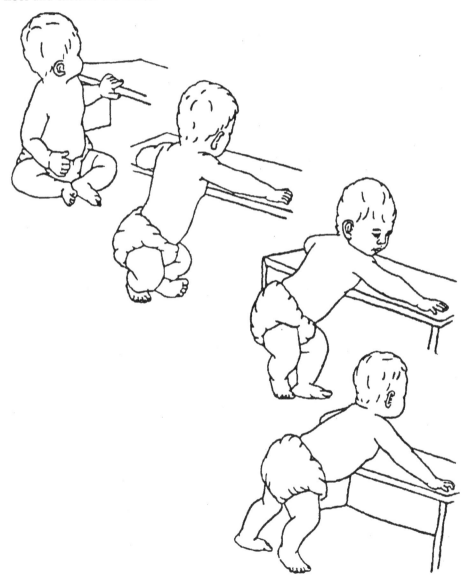

FIGURE 6.31

When first standing up, the baby may be unable to get back down and start to cry. The baby soon learns to just let go and fall down on the buttocks. When beginning to reach down to the floor for a toy, the baby develops alternate patterns to getting down (figure 6.32). Turning diagonally to the support with feet wide apart, the baby drops the pelvis back while reaching, keeping the weight more to one side. This results in an asymmetrical leg position with the inner leg more abducted and

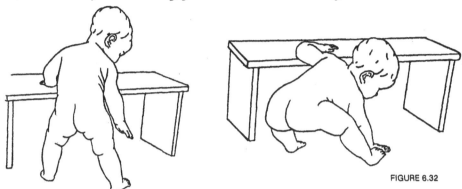

FIGURE 6.32

externally rotated and the outer leg more extended at the knee. The baby can continue to lower the buttocks to sitting and free the arms for play. With repetition, the pelvic girdle and lower extremities become more a part of the motor program for efficient movement. By the end of the ninth or tenth month, the baby begins to grade the lower extremity flexion and the descent of the pelvis is more controlled (figure 6.33). The baby may choose to shift the weight back to sitting or go forward to quadruped.

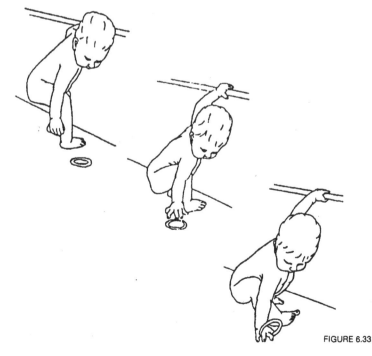

FIGURE 6.33

Standing. Initial standing may be precarious, especially if the lower extremities are not in position to provide stability for the upper body (figure 6.34). The legs may be wobbly and appear disoriented. Often the baby stands on the toes. Much of the activity at this age results in the upper body moving toward a goal and the lower extremities following. However, the baby learns to modify positions for postural stability. In standing, the baby aligns the legs under the pelvis and leans the trunk against the supporting surface. The baby also learns to adjust the posture to prepare

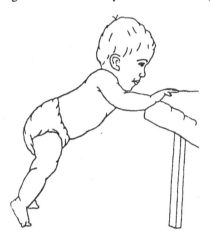

FIGURE 6.34

for functional movement. For example, the baby may be standing with adducted hips, a position that is unstable at this age for any reach or weight shift. The baby widens the base of support by taking a step sideways. Now the baby can free one arm and reach while keeping the center of gravity within the base of support (figure 6.35). Motivated to obtain objects that are out of reach, the baby uses this sidestepping pattern to cruise along furniture. This is described in greater detail in Chapter 7.

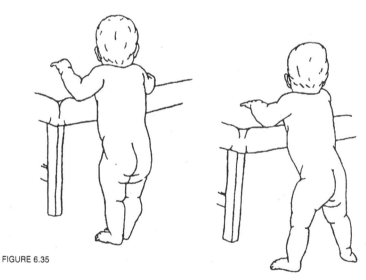

FIGURE 6.35

As balance in standing develops, the baby begins to turn the head and shoulders to visually explore the environment. Soon the baby adjusts the position of the lower body to have turned diagonal to the supporting surface (figure 6.36). At nine months of age, the baby uses this more efficient pattern to cruise along furniture. By the end of the ninth month, the baby may step from one support to another, but many babies do not accomplish this skill until the tenth or eleventh month.

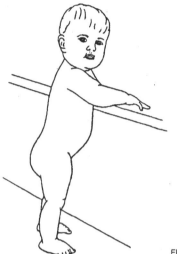

FIGURE 6.36

Pulling up on different objects, such as a coffee table, sofa, playpen, or toy box gives the child a variety of heights and surfaces of varying stability. The child learns to stand, reach, and play while adapting to the particular environment. Distal stability can be provided by leaning against a surface, weight bearing on hands or forearms, or grasping a support. The baby stands on carpet, tile, the crib mattress, and an adult's lap. Different experiences are important for learning postural control as part of the motor programs for standing. By the ninth month the baby has sufficient balance to stand with one hand held, using hip flexion and a wide base (figure 6.37).

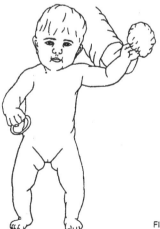

FIGURE 6.37

With two hands held, the eight-month-old child begins to walk. Although this may be a continuation of the early automatic stepping pattern of the newborn infant, the coordination is now disrupted (figure 6.38). The child lifts the leg high in the air and is unable to control the descent. The foot may land too far forward and to the side. The child may walk stiffly and on the toes, recruiting too much muscle activity. The upper body may lunge ahead of the legs. In the next month, the child begins to get control of lower extremity placement and a smooth reciprocal stepping pattern is seen.

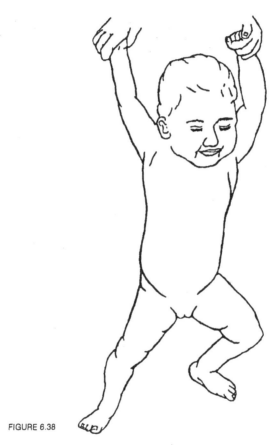

FIGURE 6.38

■ Fine Motor Development

Between seven and nine months of age, children discover that the world is "at their fingertips." Increased postural control with greater hip activity and pelvic stability allow children greater freedom to reach and move in the world. They no longer rely on adults to provide them with toys. Instead, adults must maintain a watchful eye to ensure safety as children explore new frontiers in space.

Upper Extremity Development

The child is now able to reach further in all directions and begins to understand the relationship of the body in space. During this period, the child learns how far to weight shift to obtain a toy that is beyond arm's length (figure 6.39). Due to improved hip activity, the child now can raise the arms high enough to visually examine a toy from many spatial perspectives (figure 6.40).

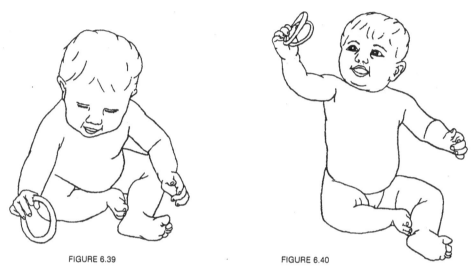

FIGURE 6.39   FIGURE 6.40

The child learns how far to bend over to reach a toy on the floor, subsequently gaining information about the whole body in relationship to space (figure 6.41). This exploration continues as the child drops objects and watches them hit the floor.

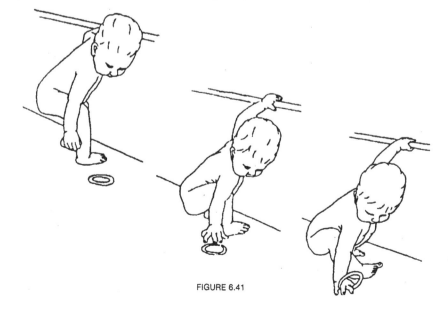

FIGURE 6.41

Control of arm function continues to improve as the child gains control of the upper extremity in weight bearing. For example, as the child rotates the trunk over an arm stabilized in weight bearing, strength and control of all muscles of the shoulder girdle is gained (figure 6.42).

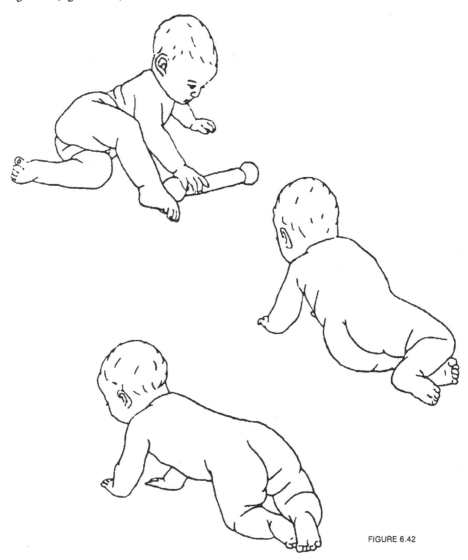

FIGURE 6.42

Scapulohumeral musculature becomes stronger, allowing the child to control humeral rotation during function. Scapulothoracic musculature is posturally challenged, thus strengthening the serratus anterior and abdominal obliques. The result of this relationship is dynamic scapular stability, which increases the child's control of the arm in space during reach and self-care. The child then can maintain the arm position in space to visually examine a toy or play So Big, wave bye-bye, and play Pat-a-Cake. As the child uses the arms to move from prone to quadruped, sidelying-to-side sit, or quadruped to stand, the muscles of the elbow, forearm, and wrist are strengthened (figure 6.43). The child then takes this postural control into function when beginning to push and pull toys. Children also begin to feed themselves, which requires dynamic control of the whole arm, trunk, hips, mouth, and eyes.

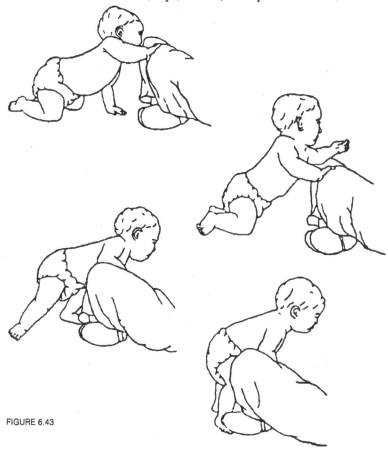

FIGURE 6.43

The child between seven to nine months of age begins to experience the potential for physical autonomy. This can be both exciting and frightening to a baby. Mentally the baby is gathering an enormous amount of information about the world. By nine months of age, the baby learns that objects are permanent. When one disappears, the baby remembers it and looks for it (Ginsberg and Opper 1969). This memory allows the baby to form emotional attachments to people and objects (White 1975). Much to the dismay of the babysitter, the baby may have a significant emotional response when a parent temporarily "disappears" for the evening. The baby remembers and searches for the parent despite the babysitter's attempts to distract the baby from the "memory." In addition, the baby pairs the concept of object permanence with sensory preferences as emotional attachments to a favorite blanket or furry stuffed animal are formed. This is not a casual relationship. These attachments are the baby's assurance that there is something constant and predictable in a world that is much larger than originally thought.

Hand Development

Experience in quadruped provides essential input to the hand as the child rocks back and forth, uses transitions, and creeps. This transfer of weight lengthens the muscles and soft tissue in the palm and fingers. As the child moves in and out of quadruped and side sitting, balance reactions develop in the hand, reinforcing the palmar arches (Boehme 1988). The deep sensory input experienced in weight bearing prepares the child between seven and nine months of age to develop higher-level prehension patterns.

The child has a strong grip and can maintain an object against resistance (figure 6.44). This requires strength in all the muscles of the arm and shoulder as well as stability in the trunk. This full body control is demonstrated in the precision of the child's reach and grasp (figures 6.45 and 6.46). The child's movements are directed by fully developed vision and the cognitive ability to focus attention on the task at hand.

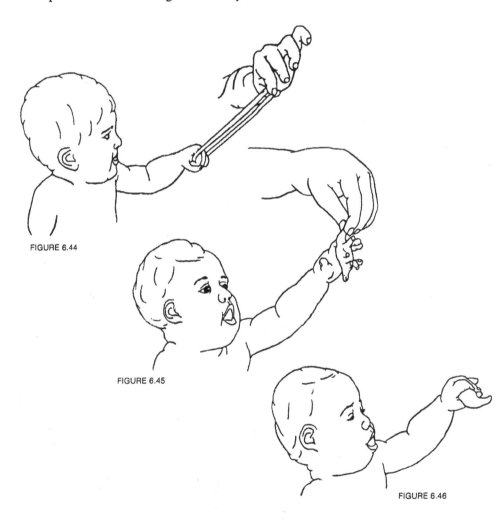

FIGURE 6.44

FIGURE 6.45

FIGURE 6.46

The seven-month-old baby is mastering the radial-palmar grasp and can now supinate the forearm to visually explore the reverse side of toys (figure 6.47). Supination requires control of the shoulder, elbow, and wrist, developed in dynamic, transitional, gross motor activity. At eight months of age, the child uses a radial-digital grasp where the object is held with an opposed thumb and fingertips (Erhardt 1982). The space visible between the thumb and fingers indicates that the palmar arches are active (figure 6.48). By nine months of age, the wrist is initially positioned in neutral and then in extension. These new prehension patterns as well as more primitive ones are used in play.

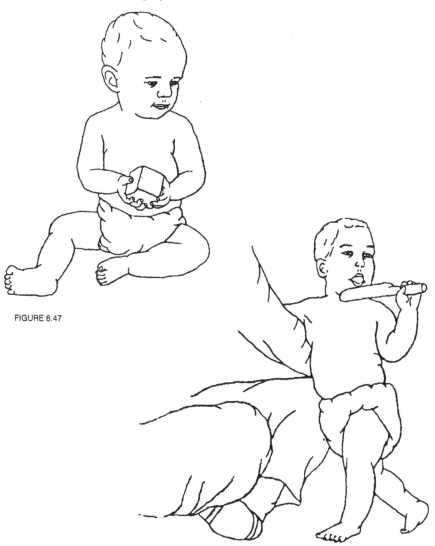

FIGURE 6.47

FIGURE 6.48

The child often obtains a toy and carries it while creeping across the carpet (figure 6.49). This weight bearing over the ulnar side of the hand helps the child develop dissociation between the ulnar and radial sides of the hand. Once the two sides of the hand begin to work independently of each other, the child uses finer prehension

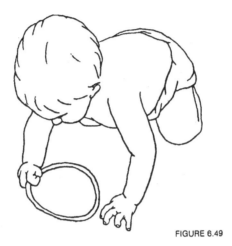

FIGURE 6.49

patterns, such as the three-jaw chuck (figure 6.50) and index finger pointing (figure 6.51). The child is progressing toward pinch, beginning with raking at seven months of age, where he uses the fingers to draw small objects into the palm. A lateral pinch is used at eight months and an inferior pinch emerges at nine months, when the child obtains the object between the thumb and mid ventral surface of the index finger (figure 6.52) (Hohlstein 1982).

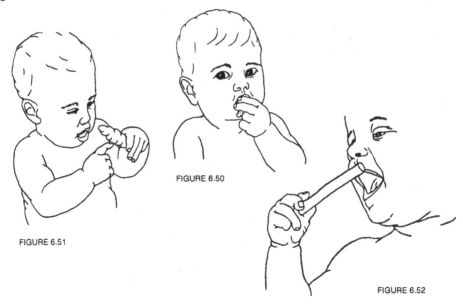

FIGURE 6.50

FIGURE 6.51

FIGURE 6.52

Progressively between seven and nine months, the child learns to release objects, first by releasing them against a surface and then, by nine months, releasing them in midair (Erhardt 1982). The child can also successfully release an object into a large container, gaining more information about size, shape, and depth.

In addition, improved hip and trunk control give the child freedom to easily explore an object with two hands and to explore the hands as the total focus of interest (figure 6.53). The child can play with an object in each hand and drop one object to obtain another. The child utilizes combinations of all the upper extremity patterns thus far developed as self-care skills are initiated. The child bottlefeeds himself or herself effortlessly, using control of humeral rotation, midrange elbow flexion, neutral forearm rotation with wrist extension, and an expanded, controlled hand (figure 6.54). The child finger feeds with less grace, using the jaw as a base of stability for finer function (figure 6.55). The child is also eager to assist with spoonfeeding and cupdrinking (figures 6.56 and 6.57). Functional activity becomes more than an interesting sensory experience. It now incorporates a cognitive goal and an anticipated result.

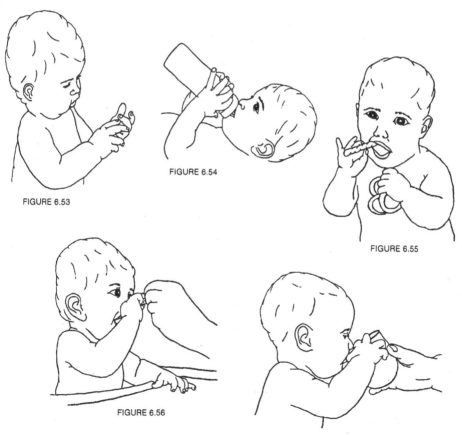

FIGURE 6.54

FIGURE 6.53

FIGURE 6.55

FIGURE 6.56

FIGURE 6.57

■ Oral-Motor and Respiratory Development

Anatomical/Structural Characteristics

The oral and pharyngeal mechanisms. Modifications in the contour, shape, size, and alignment of the structures and musculature of the oral and pharyngeal mechanisms as described in Chapters 4 and 5 continue from seven through nine months of age.

Rib cage and diaphragm. The downwardly rotated contour and alignment of the rib cage and the more elongated chest wall reflect the baby's increased experience with postural control in more upright positions and greater use of the abdominal musculature with improved pelvic and hip control in movement (figure 6.58). As the abdominal musculature becomes more active, providing more consistent downward stability to the rib cage and more support for the structures of the abdominal cavity, greater intra-abdominal pressure is created. This results in more effective contraction of the diaphragm during inhalation (Massery 1991).

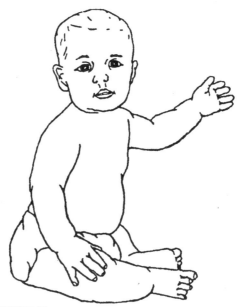

FIGURE 6.58

Although belly breathing continues to be predominant, the baby begins to exhibit some active rib cage expansion on inhalation. Downward rotation of the ribs by gravity and abdominal musculature activity is creating a widening of the spaces between the ribs and preparation of the intercostal muscles for function during inhalation and exhalation. As the intercostal muscles gradually become more active, the baby's rib cage has greater internal stability and begins to exhibit active upward and outward expansion during inhalation.

Developmental Characteristics

From seven to nine months of age, babies investigate new objects in their environment by obtaining information through a variety of sensory channels. They continue to use the oral mechanism for exploration, but are now combining this in a more organized manner with visual examination and manipulation of the objects (figure 6.59).

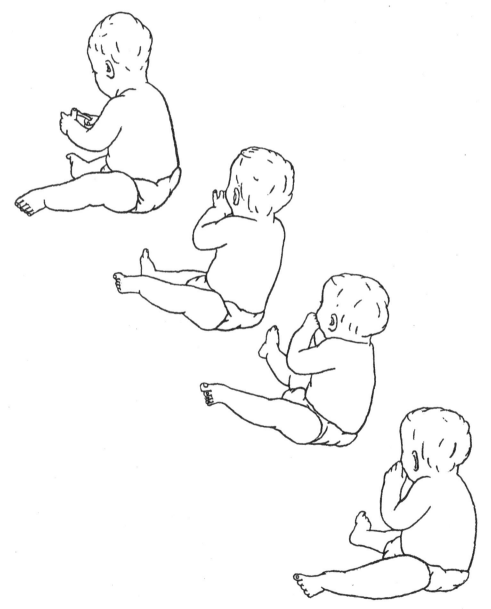

FIGURE 6.59

Teething continues to influence the baby's need to bring fingers and hard objects into the mouth for biting. The primary reason for this activity is to relieve some of the discomfort felt as the gums swell and the teeth erupt through the gum tissue. However, this biting activity also provides greater experience in jaw and tongue movements separate from the feeding process. Sucking on the thumb or fingers may be used more often as the baby attempts to become calm or quiet when fatigued or stressed (figure 6.60).

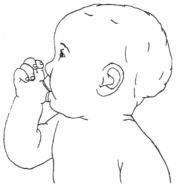

FIGURE 6.60

Improved postural control and more coordinated head, neck, shoulder girdle, trunk, pelvis, and hip musculature activity in movement free the child to experience more active and coordinated jaw, tongue, and lip movements in supine, prone, sitting, and standing (figures 6.61 and 6.62). The child is learning to coordinate and organize oral-motor movements on a more secure and stable foundation of postural activity. Drooling rarely occurs except when teething.

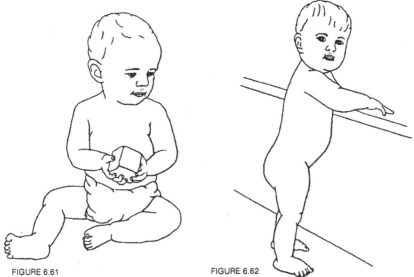

FIGURE 6.61   FIGURE 6.62

When involved in newer gross motor activities such as quadruped, creeping on hands and knees, and pulling-to-stand, the baby generally produces fewer, less coordinated movements of the oral mechanism. This is also evident when the baby is focused on new upper extremity tasks (figure 6.63). Increased drooling may be noted at these times when oral-motor activity is minimal and the child is intensely focused on these new gross motor and upper extremity experiences.

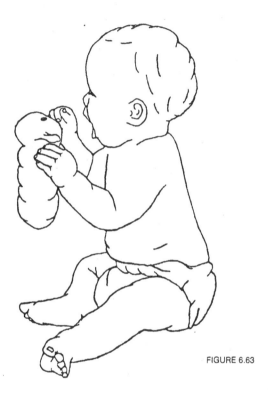

FIGURE 6.63

The feeding process. From seven to nine months of age, children are developing new jaw, tongue, and lip movements as well as more coordinated oral-motor activity. They are learning to organize and coordinate their new oral movements with pharyngeal, respiratory, and postural activity during a variety of feeding and drinking tasks.

The seven-month-old child generally sits in a highchair or infant seat for feeding with the seat back positioned at a 90-degree angle. Adaptations are required that help support the baby posturally. Parents often use restrainer vests, pillows, or a tray to provide the external supports needed during feeding.

By nine months of age, the baby has developed adequate postural control in sitting to maintain this position in the highchair without vests or pillows for external support. Seat belts and trays are used for safety reasons rather than being needed for positional support.

During bottledrinking and breastfeeding, the mouth is opened and a quiet jaw and tongue position is maintained as the nipple is brought toward and inserted in the mouth. Sucking is the predominant oral-motor pattern used by the baby (figure 6.64). The lips, cheeks, jaw, and tongue are well organized in their movements, resulting in long sequences of coordinated sucking, swallowing, and breathing activity. Suckling movements of the oral mechanism may still be noted, but on a very limited basis. By nine months of age, the child no longer loses liquid when sucking is initiated on the nipple or when the nipple is removed from the mouth. Oral and pharyngeal function during bottledrinking and breastfeeding is characterized by efficient, well-coordinated activity.

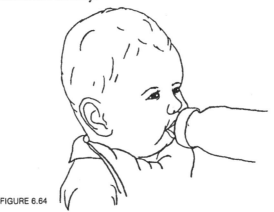

FIGURE 6.64

Rhythmical forward/backward movements of the tongue, wide up/down excursions of the jaw, and minimal lip activity characteristic of suckling are predominant during cupdrinking from seven to nine months of age. When the adult holds the cup firmly in the infant's mouth, more coordinated sucking movements of the jaw, tongue, and lips may be experienced. However, cup removal, repositioning, or reinsertion results in the loss of this more coordinated oral activity and the return to suckling with a significant loss of liquid.

Cups with spouted lids are extremely popular ways to present liquid (figure 6.65). The spout provides a stability point for the child within the mouth during drinking, limits the amount of liquid entering the mouth, and keeps spillage to a minimum.

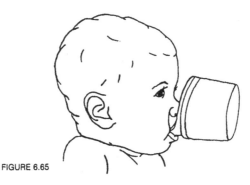

FIGURE 6.65

However, most babies do not receive liquid exclusively through the spouted cup. They still experience cupdrinking with a regular cup. This provides the sensory-motor experiences required for future development of the well-coordinated tongue, jaw, and lip movements that are necessary for controlling liquid in the mouth and guiding the liquid posteriorly in swallowing.

Problems in coordinating sucking/suckling, swallowing, and breathing persist at seven months of age during cupdrinking. The baby may continuously suck or suckle, bringing more liquid into the mouth than can actually be handled. An attempt to swallow the liquid generally results in coughing and choking, with most of the liquid lost from the mouth. If the mouthful is too large, the baby may just let it flow out of the mouth without attempting to swallow. Although coordinating sucking/suckling, swallowing, and breathing is still difficult by nine months of age, the baby has learned to control the activity by taking fewer sucks/suckles (1 to 3) at a time before pulling away from the cup to breathe (figures 6.66).

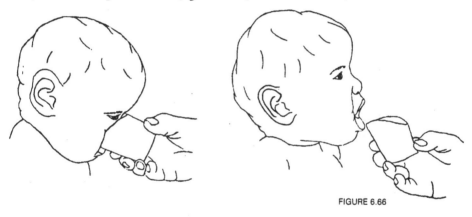

FIGURE 6.66

The seven-month-old baby begins to use the upper lip more actively in the spoonfeeding process. The upper lip moves forward and downward to posture on the spoon as it enters the mouth (figures 6.67 and 6.68). As the spoon is being removed, the upper lip begins to move inward, assisting in the removal process (figure 6.69). This forward, downward, and inward sequence of upper lip movement in spoonfeeding continues to increase in its use over the next few months.

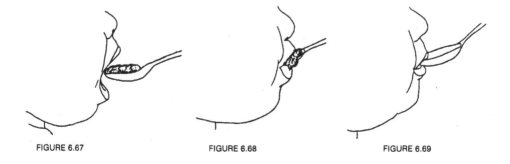

FIGURE 6.67   FIGURE 6.68   FIGURE 6.69

From seven through nine months of age, children are using a mixture of sucking and suckling movements of the tongue, jaw, cheeks, and lips to handle semisolids. They are being introduced to new textures such as junior foods, ground foods, and some carefully mashed table foods in addition to the pureed foods they have already been receiving. New textures may initially stimulate some gagging and choking, but the baby quickly learns to adjust to these new sensory experiences. When swallowing and clearing semisolids from the oropharyngeal area, the baby may still use some forward/backward tongue movements and easy tongue protrusion as well as some emerging up/down tongue activity. At eight to nine months of age, active lip closure occurs more often as part of the swallowing process (Stolovitz and Gisel 1991).

New oral-motor activity is emerging over the seven- to nine-month period as babies gain experience in biting and chewing with soft and hard solids. Phasic up/down movements of the jaw continue to be seen when a hard solid is placed in the mouth (figure 6.70). Although not yet able to bite through a soft cookie, by nine months of age the child stabilizes the jaw in a closed position and holds it closed on the cookie until a piece is broken off (figure 6.71).

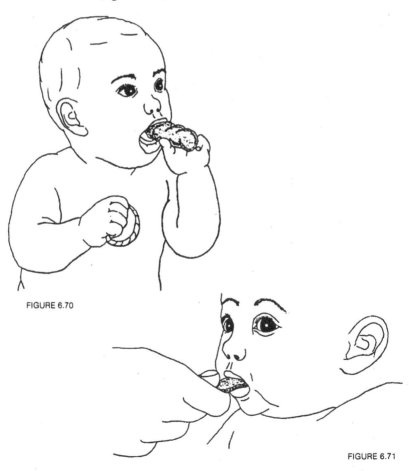

FIGURE 6.70

FIGURE 6.71

During chewing, jaw movements are primarily up and down in direction with significant variability in regard to the width of their excursions. Lateral movements of the tongue and diagonal movements of the jaw occur when food is placed directly on the side biting surfaces. As the tongue begins to transfer food from the center of the mouth to the side for chewing, the nine-month-old baby begins to move the jaw in a diagonal and circular motion, which may be referred to as diagonal rotary pattern (figure 6.72) (Morris and Klein 1987). The lips move actively in direct relationship to the jaw movements (figure 6.73). Tongue protrusion and forward/backward tongue movements still occur as part of the swallowing process.

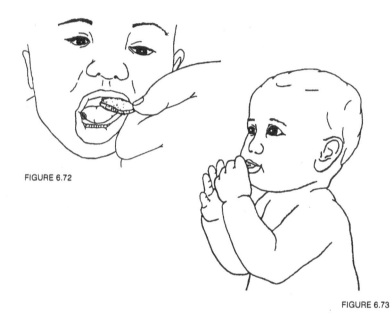

FIGURE 6.72

FIGURE 6.73

Significant changes are also occurring in regard to the child's integration of new head/neck, trunk, hip, and upper extremity/hand activities during feeding. The bottle is often held by the baby during bottledrinking. The baby comes forward with the trunk over the hips and flexes the head downward to assist during cupdrinking and spoonfeeding (figure 6.74). Newly emerging prehension patterns and greater

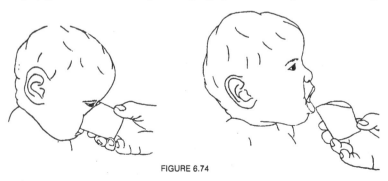

FIGURE 6.74

postural control allow the child to bring solids such as cookies, pieces of cereal, and teething biscuits to the mouth for fingerfeeding (figures 6.75 and 6.76). The baby is becoming an extremely active participant in all aspects of feeding.

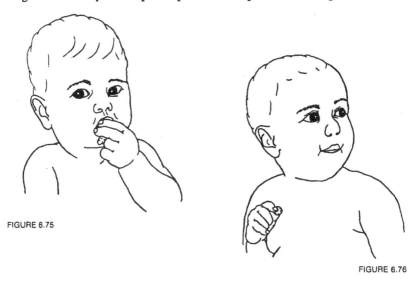

FIGURE 6.75

FIGURE 6.76

Significant components of respiratory function. As the baby uses the abdominal musculature, specifically the abdominal obliques, more actively in movement with a base of greater active postural control, significant changes in respiratory function begin to emerge (figure 6.77). A more mature respiratory pattern with anterior and lateral expansion of the rib cage may occur on inhalation when the baby is posturally

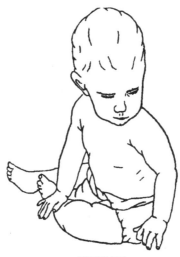

FIGURE 6.77

active and stable (figure 6.78). Rib flaring is gradually becoming less evident during belly breathing as the abdominal obliques more effectively stabilize the lower rib cage in coordination with the contraction of the diaphragm. Increasing abdominal musculature activity and strength provide a foundation from which the external and internal intercostals are prepared for active function and from which diaphragmatic activity can be more effective and efficient. These factors, among others, not only influence changes in the structures and alignment of the respiratory mechanism, but also in the coordination of respiration with all functional activities the infant is learning to perform. Although use of an efficient adult abdominal-thoracic breathing pattern is years in the future, the musculature activity and structural changes emerging in the seven- to nine-month period set the stage for its development (Davis 1987).

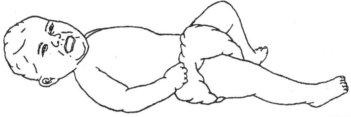

FIGURE 6.78

By eight to nine months of age, the child begins to produce sounds separate from active body movements. More integrated musculature activity and greater internal postural control provide a foundation from which better respiratory control and coordination with laryngeal and oral activity can be produced. Babies continue to play with sound productions during gross motor and upper extremity activities (figure 6.79). However, they no longer need to be actively moving through their bodies to generate sufficient musculature activity to support their production of sounds.

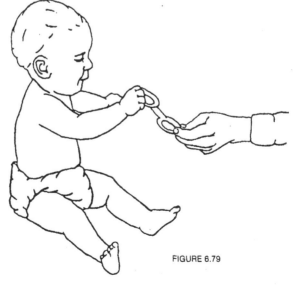

FIGURE 6.79

Babies now produce longer chains of repeated consonant-vowel combinations (reduplicated babbling) as they have adequate support from the respiratory musculature and sufficient air intake to produce phonation of greater duration. Syllables are more adult-like in their length and more rhythmical in their speed of production. Consonants produced with lip-to-lip contact (bilabials) and tongue-to-alveolar ridge contact (lingual-alveolars) are becoming more prevalent. Greater differentiation between nasal and oral sounds produced at the same place of articulatory contact (for example, /b/ and /m/; /d/ and /n/) can be heard in the child's babbling, reflecting greater control of the musculature of the soft palate for velopharyngeal closure during sound production. This is a time when parents often perceive certain consonant-vowel combinations produced by the child as being the first words (for example, /dɑdɑ/ for Daddy). See Chapter 8 for further information on sound production development.

Summary Chart–7-9 Months

Postural Control	Gross Motor	Reach	Fine Motor
Equilibrium reactions present in prone and supine (7 months), in sitting and beginning in quadruped (8 months)	Increased use of sidelying as a position for play with greater variety of postures; moves from sidelying to quadruped	Upper extremities free for bilateral play such as So Big, Pat-A-Cake, and Peek-A-Boo	Demonstrates grip strength
Protective extension of the arms sideways in sitting (8 months)	Sits on floor without arm support • able to move upper body over base of support to reach and play • uses a variety of postures including side-sitting • moves from sitting to prone • transitions between sitting and quadruped	Reaches further in all directions due to increasing postural control	Masters radial–palmar grasp
Increased postural activity to • maintain upright positions • accompany functional movement in sitting, quadruped, and standing at a support • transition between sitting, quadruped, and supported standing	Maintains quadruped • rocks forward and back • reaches in all directions • modifies position by weight bearing on one or both feet rather than on knees • transitions to sidelying, sitting, and kneeling with support	Uses upper extremities to move body into higher positions in gravity	Develops radial-digital grasp
Increased ability to adapt posture prior to a movement for more efficient execution	Pivots sideways and belly crawls in prone		Points; is developing a pinch
	Creeps reciprocally on hands and knees using lateral flexion/elongation pattern of trunk; may creep on hands, knee, and foot or on hands and feet		Releases objects in space and into large containers
	Kneels at supporting surface with hip flexion, greater hip extension by 9 months • sits back on heels to play • uses as part of transition to standing		Independently bottle feeds
	Pulls to standing at supported surface using mostly arms and upper body • leans against support and plays • lowers self to floor		Continues to fingerfeed
	Cruises along furniture • initially steps sideways • learns to turn diagonal to support and step forward		Assists with cup and spoonfeeding
	Stands with one hand held; begins to walk with two hands held in uncoordinated pattern		

Some infants develop activities earlier or later than this chart indicates. Therefore, it should not be regarded as a rigid timetable of events.

Summary Chart—7-9 Months continued

Oral-Motor/Feeding	Respiration-Phonation
Gag response diminishes in strength to a more adult protective gag response	*Respiration* Belly breathing with greater belly expansion on inhalation; less rib flaring occurs
Feeding Sucks liquid from bottle/breast with no liquid loss and long sequences of coordinated sucking-swallowing-breathing; no loss of liquid on nipple insertion/removal (9 months)	Anterior/lateral expansion of rib cage may occur on inhalation during crying or when posturally active and stable (8-9 months)
Suckles liquid presented by cup • brings lower lip up under cup and sucks in liquid when cup is held firmly in mouth • loses liquid with cup removal, repositioning, or reinsertion • coughs/chokes when takes in too much liquid • takes fewer sucks/suckles before pulling away from cup to breathe (9 months)	Coordinates breathing more easily with general movement, feeding, swallowing, and sound production
Uses variable up/down jaw movements in chewing • moves tongue laterally and jaw diagonally with solids placed on side biting surfaces • as tongue transfers food center to side, jaw moves in diagonal-circular motion (9 months) • lips move actively with jaw • uses tongue protrusion and forward/backward tongue movements on the swallow	*Phonation/Sounds* Produces phonation/sounds separate from active body movement (8-9 months)
Oral-Motor Uses facial expressions that convey likes/dislikes	Produces long chains of repeated consonant-vowel combinations (reduplicated babbling)
Uses mouth to investigate new objects in combination with visual examination and hand manipulation	Begins producing consonants with lip-to-lip and tongue-to-alveolar ridge contact
Bites on fingers/objects to reduce teething discomfort	Produces/differentiates nasal and oral sounds with same place of articulation contact (/b/ and /m/; /d/ and /n/)
Sucks on thumb/fingers to calm/quiet/organize	Produces consonant-vowel combinations that may be perceived by adult as a word (/dɑdɑ/ for daddy)
Produces more coordinated jaw, tongue, and lip movements in supine, prone, sitting, and standing; drooling rarely occurs except when teething	
May posture mouth for stability or produce less oral activity when in quadruped, creeping on hands and knees, pulling to stand, and involved in new upper extremity activities; may drool	

Opens/quiets mouth as spoon approaches
• brings lower lip up under spoon
• moves upper lip forward, down, and inward to remove food from spoon
• uses a mixture of sucking and suckling to move food back
• uses tongue protrusion as well as forward/backward and some up/down tongue movements on the swallow
• may close lips on the swallow (9 months)
• may gag/choke on new textures

Uses phasic up/down jaw movements on hard solids; holds jaw closed on soft solid until piece is broken off (9 months)

■ References

Boehme, R. 1988. *Improving upper body control.* Tucson, AZ: Therapy Skill Builders.

Davis, L. F. 1987. Respiration and phonation in cerebral palsy: A developmental model. *Seminars in Speech and Language* 8(1):101-06.

Erhardt, R. P. 1982. *Developmental hand dysfunction: Theory, assessment, and treatment.* Tucson, AZ: Therapy Skill Builders.

Ginsburg, H., and S. Opper. 1969. *Piaget's theory of intellectual development: An introduction.* Englewood Cliffs, NJ: Prentice Hall.

Hohlstein, R. 1982. The development of prehension in normal infants. *The American Journal of Occupational Therapy* 36(3):170-76.

Massery, M. 1991. Chest development as a component of normal motor development: Implications for pediatric physical therapists. *Pediatric Physical Therapy* 3(1):3-8.

Morris, S. E., and M. D. Klein. 1987. *Pre-Feeding skills.* Tucson, AZ: Therapy Skill Builders.

Stolovitz, P., and E. Gisel. 1991. Circumoral movements in response to three different food textures in children 6 months to 2 years of age. *Dysphagia* 6:17-25.

White, B. 1975. *The first three years of life.* Englewood Cliffs, NJ: Prentice Hall.

Chapter 7

10-12 Months

■ Postural Control

The child's ability to maintain an upright posture becomes more efficient and functional in this last trimester as postural stability of the lower body further develops. The lumbar spine extends through a greater range in sitting, kneeling, and standing, allowing the upper body to be vertically aligned over the pelvis and hips. The S-curve of the spinal column is seen more consistently, providing mechanical as well as muscular stability for postural alignment. This pattern together with other lower body activity frees the lower extremities from postures that mechanically stabilize the base of support (abduction/external rotation of the hips). From 10 to 12 months of age the baby is able to sit, kneel, and stand with support, using a more mature pattern of postural control. For example, lumbar extension enables the baby to side-sit with the upper extremities free for play (figure 7.1). In kneeling and

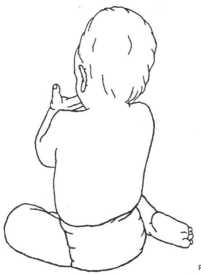

FIGURE 7.1

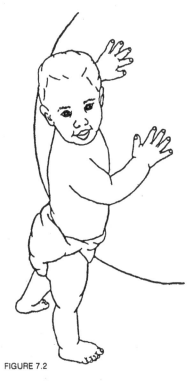

FIGURE 7.2

standing with support, the arms are used only as a distal point of stability for balance. Because the head and shoulders are more directly over the hip joint rather than anterior, the baby no longer needs to lean on the upper extremities (figure 7.2). However, independent standing and walking still require positional stability of the lower extremities, especially external rotation of the hip.

In addition to increased extension of the lumbar spine, the baby also uses more muscle activity of the lower extremities to maintain postures, especially during upper extremity function. In sitting, the quadriceps may extend the knee to stabilize the leg as the hands are used for fine motor activities. The ankle and foot musculature more intensely activate, providing distal stability during reach and play. Also, the weight-bearing foot is more active against the surface in sitting and standing. The toes, in particular, demonstrate an increased level of participation. They flex, extend, or abduct to help stabilize the foot and leg during sitting activities. In weight bearing, the toes can flex to grasp the surface or extend to push against the floor. The latter is seen clearly in standing as the baby goes up on the toes when using the arms for play at a supporting surface (figure 7.3).

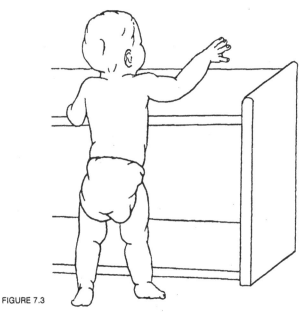

FIGURE 7.3

Pelvic and lower extremity activity not only contribute to maintenance of postures, but also play an important role in the development of coordination of posture with movement. Although beginning to shift weight in prone through pelvic girdle activity at six months of age, the baby initiated movement in more upright positions from the head and upper body. In sitting and quadruped, the baby now begins to displace the center of gravity by moving the pelvis over the femurs during weight shifts. In sitting, the baby can move the pelvis in all planes, forward/backward, lateral, and around the vertical axis (rotation). In this way the baby can shift the center of gravity in wider ranges while reaching and can move in and out of a variety of sitting postures.

The baby can also more efficiently change position by moving the center of gravity throughout the entire transition. For example, when moving from sit to quadruped, the eight-month-old child first rotated the head and upper trunk and placed the arms in a position to accept weight. Then, leaning over the hip, the child used a forward momentum to move the center of gravity into a new position. The 10- or 11-month-old child begins the movement by rotating the pelvis over the femur, shifting the center of gravity to initiate the transition. The child continues to control the movement as the spine rotates progressively upward and the body moves forward over the arms. In addition to pelvic motion, the foot is able to push against the floor to aid in moving the center of gravity during transitions. This occurs when the baby stands up with support from half-kneeling or from squat in the middle of the room as well as during other transitions.

Postural reactions to an unexpected movement of the center of gravity continue to develop in this last trimester. Protective extension of the arms is present backwards in sitting by 10 months of age. Equilibrium reactions can be elicited in quadruped and are more refined in sitting. They are beginning in kneeling and standing with support. Spontaneous postural reactions occur less often in sitting and quadruped than in previous months because postural accompaniments are more adequately coordinated with movement in these positions. However, they are frequently seen as the baby begins independent standing and walking. By 18 months of age the baby learns to more efficiently coordinate postural control and movement for ambulation on smooth surfaces and seldom falls.

■ Gross Motor Development

The 10- to 12-month-old child is busy exploring the surroundings in more upright positions. Moving easily in and out of a variety of positions during play, the baby experiments with posture and movement while learning about the environment. Much time is spent pulling to standing, cruising, and lowering the body back down to the floor. Quieter babies may just now begin to sit independently and creep, but they learn these skills together with standing in a short period of time. By the end of the first year, the baby is able to sequence many different movement patterns and begins upright locomotion.

Sitting. During these three months, sitting becomes a more dynamic and functional position as postural control and mobility continue to develop. Pelvic motion increases, partially due to greater pelvic-femoral mobility. In particular, the range of hip internal rotation increases. The hips and lower extremities become more posturally active, including the foot that is used dynamically as a point of distal stability. Weight shift can be initiated and controlled through pelvic girdle activity. These factors allow the baby to use an even greater variety of sitting postures than was used in the previous months.

The more dynamic role of the lower extremities in sitting is clearly demonstrated by the use of the foot against the floor as part of the base of support (figure 7.4). Before this, the baby sat with portions of the lateral or posterior aspects of the upper and lower leg touching the floor, but now can use only the foot as the point of contact. Although using this position for transitions, the seven- to nine-month-old baby was unable to maintain it for play. The hip and foot control the position of the upper and lower leg in space, with varying degrees of knee flexion (see figure 7.10a, page 179). This lower extremity ability contributes to a more efficient weight shift and reach in a wide range.

Another dynamic lower extremity pattern is seen as the baby sits with active extension of one knee (figure 7.5). The quadriceps muscle is contracting and the foot is usually plantar flexed with the toes curled. Depending on the activity and direction of weight shift, the hip can be held in neutral or in some degree of rotation. The biomechanics

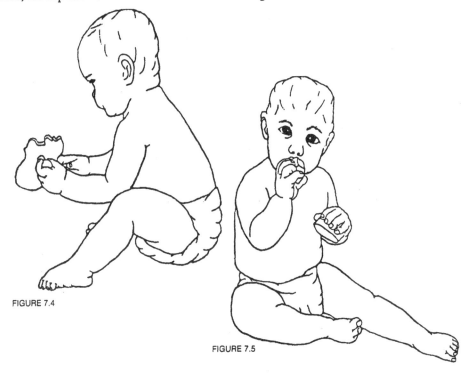

FIGURE 7.4

FIGURE 7.5

of the pattern may limit full knee extension. For example, external rotation of the hip requires more elongation of the hamstrings so the knee will flex slightly as the musculature reaches its maximum length. The 12-month-old baby begins to "long sit" with both knees extended but slightly externally rotated.

Increased mobility of the hip into internal rotation with flexion makes it possible for the baby to W-sit (figure 7.6). This is different from heel-sitting in which the hips are in neutral rotation and the feet are under the buttocks. In W-sitting the hips are in the end range of internal rotation with the pelvis between the feet. The ankles are usually plantar flexed. The baby assumes this position in a number of ways. Commonly, the baby internally rotates the femurs when sitting back from quadruped or lowering the pelvis from squat during transitioning from standing to the floor. W-sitting provides a stable posture for lateral reach (figure 7.7) and an easy transition to creeping.

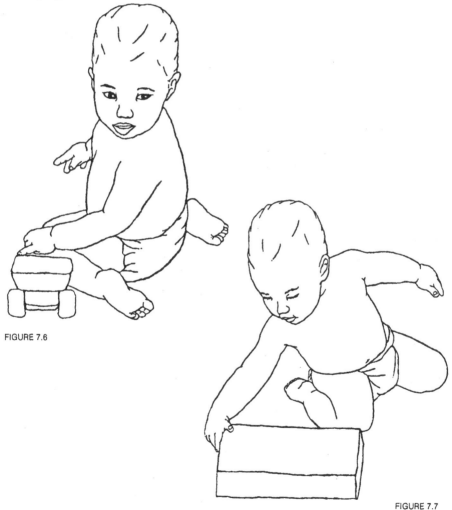

FIGURE 7.6

FIGURE 7.7

The baby is also able to sit with one leg internally rotated in the same pattern as W-sitting and the other leg externally rotated (figure 7.8). This position allows greater trunk rotation for reach or when transitioning to another position. The baby often assumes this posture by moving forward over the legs to reach a toy and then sitting back. As the baby shifts the weight forward, the pelvis rises off the surface and one hip internally rotates as a postural accompaniment. When the baby moves back and lowers the buttocks to the floor, the hip remains internally rotated.

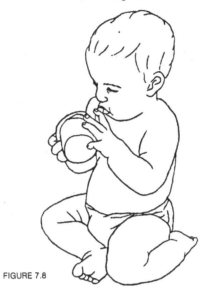

FIGURE 7.8

Another variation in this posture occurs when the baby has one foot on the floor in quadruped and internally rotates the opposite hip while lowering the pelvis. Now the baby sits with one leg in the W pattern and the other knee up with the foot on the floor (figure 7.9). This pattern offers an easy transition back to quadruped. The baby may also use this pattern when transitioning between supported standing and sitting on the floor.

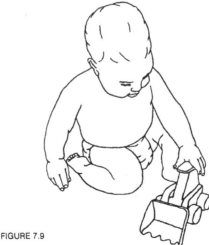

FIGURE 7.9

Activity of the foot is important to the development of the various sitting postures in the 10- to 12-month period. Through weight bearing, the foot provides stability for proximal activity and helps control the position of the lower leg while biomechanically influencing the femur. As the baby plays, the foot provides distal stability for weight shifts through the pelvis and hips. The ankle may be dorsiflexed so only the heel is in contact with the floor (figure 7.10a) or it may be plantar flexed allowing the forefoot to push against the surface (figure 7.10b).

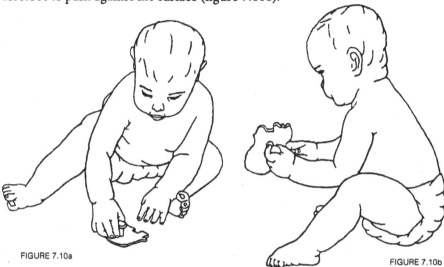

FIGURE 7.10a

FIGURE 7.10b

The foot is also active in nonweight-bearing patterns. When the knee is extended, the foot contributes to stability through ankle dorsiflexion or plantar flexion. Inversion and eversion of the foot is also seen in combination with dorsiflexion or plantar flexion. Inversion often occurs with hip external rotation (figure 7.10c) and eversion with internal rotation (figure 7.10d).

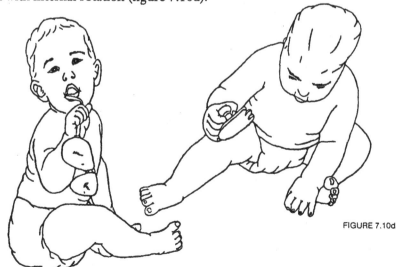

FIGURE 7.10d

FIGURE 7.10c

Increased postural activity is also seen in the toes in various patterns. The long toe flexors can be activated with either dorsiflexion (see figure 7.10d) or plantar flexion (see figure 7.10b). The long toe extensors may stabilize the toes in an extended position and also evert the foot (see figure 7.10a). Since the great toe has its own musculature, it can flex or extend independent of the other toes (figure 7.10e). Abduction of the great toe often accompanies inversion of the foot (see figure 7.10c).

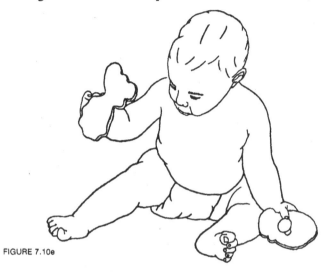

FIGURE 7.10e

The baby's ability to control movement of the center of gravity in wider ranges contributes to a functional sitting position. Increased mobility and further development of postural control allow the baby to move the center of gravity by shifting the weight from the lower extremity, hip, and pelvis rather than through the shoulder girdle and upper trunk. The baby can move the center of gravity forward by flexing the hips while extending the spine (figure 7.11). Increased hip mobility allows the

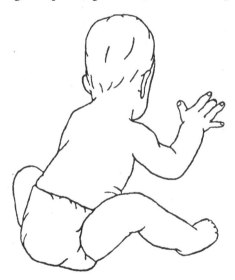

FIGURE 7.11

pelvis to move forward between abducted femurs. When shifting the weight back, an active posterior tilt of the pelvis occurs rather than the trunk sinking into flexion (figure 7.12). This requires abdominal control in synergy with spinal extensors and the base of the pelvis working against the floor. Some babies have enough postural control in this posture to kick their legs reciprocally or to lift one foot and pull off a sock.

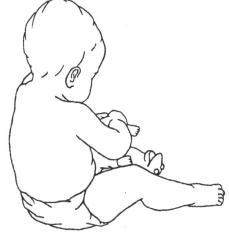

FIGURE 7.12

The baby also shifts the weight laterally onto one hip through pelvic girdle activity and maintains that position while playing (figure 7.13). When rotating the spine in sitting, the baby can initiate the movement from the pelvis and progressively rotate the intervertebral joints from the lumbar-sacral area upward. Before this, the rotation was initiated from the head and shoulders and progressed downward. The weight can be shifted to the hip opposite the side the baby is turning to (see figure 7.10c, page 179) or to the same side. Both movements involve the pelvis rotating over the femur, which is kinesiological internal or external rotation of the hip. Lateral weight shift and rotation require active stability of the more weight-bearing hip against the floor.

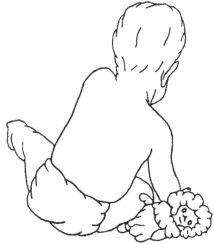

FIGURE 7.13

The ability to move and control the center of gravity through more pelvic and lower extremity activity allows the baby to obtain objects in a wider range of the environment without transitioning to another position. For example, instead of moving forward to quadruped and reaching, the baby leans the pelvis forward and pushes the abducted/externally rotated leg against the floor, lifting the buttocks just enough to reach the object (figure 7.14). The opposite leg can be internally rotated and flexed at the hip and knee or extended to the side (figure 7.15).

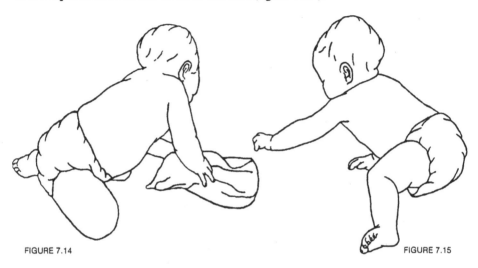

FIGURE 7.14   FIGURE 7.15

To obtain an object located at one side, the baby can use several options. The baby can flex and rotate the pelvis over one hip (relative internal rotation) and push on the arm to move the center of gravity forward (figure 7.16). The opposite leg provides a counterbalance through external rotation of the hip and stability of the foot on the floor. If the object is further away, the baby shifts the center of gravity so the pelvis rises off the floor. Pivoting around the weight-bearing hip, the baby now sits with one

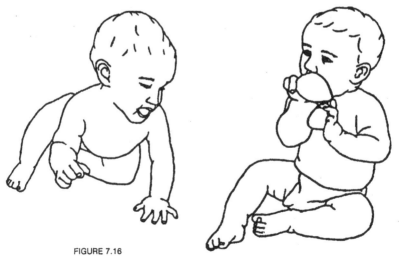

FIGURE 7.16

leg internally rotated and the other externally rotated (figure 7.17). Another option is demonstrated in figure 7.18. The extended knee provides stability as the baby shifts the weight over one hip and lifts the opposite leg in the air. The baby then flexes the extended knee and pushes that leg and the hand against the floor, raising the pelvis. The nonweight-bearing hip externally rotates and the foot is planted on the floor. The baby reaches for the toy and returns to a sitting position.

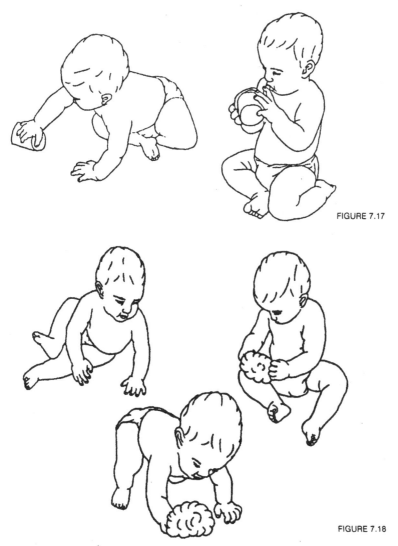

FIGURE 7.17

FIGURE 7.18

To interact with an object in the environment, the baby has a choice of several postures. Motor learning requires experimentation. Through trial and error the baby learns how to orientate the body toward an object, the direction to shift weight, and the postural control necessary to accompany the reach. Additionally, the baby must learn to coordinate the reach itself as well as the grasp and manipulation of the object.

By 12 months of age, sitting becomes an extremely functional position for reach and play. The child can use a variety of patterns in succession (figure 7.19). First, using one foot on the floor, the child moves forward to obtain a puzzle piece and then sits back on the opposite heel to examine it. The child can easily obtain a second piece by internally rotating that hip and externally rotating the opposite leg. The child extends the internally rotated leg in front of the body for a more symmetrical stable base of support and bangs the two pieces together. The ability to sequence various sitting postures plays an important role in early perceptual/cognitive development.

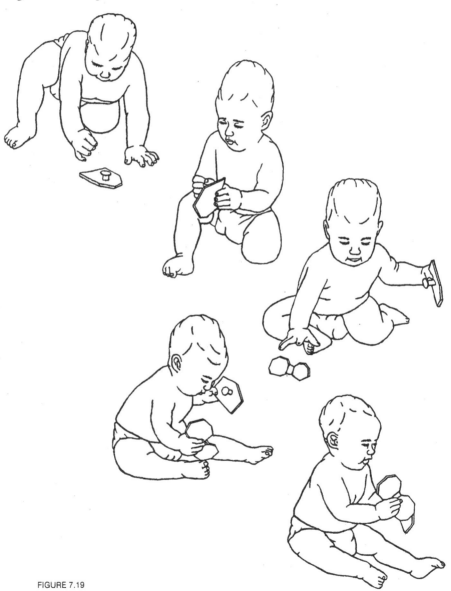

FIGURE 7.19

In addition to floor sitting, the child is also capable of sitting independently on a small stool or chair. The child might enjoy sitting on a rocking or riding toy without support but probably still needs help to get on and off it. Although sitting balance is well developed, safety belts are still important in strollers and shopping carts because the child now tries to stand up or climb out of them.

Transitions in and out of sitting. Sometime in the 10- to 12-month period, the baby learns to sit up from sidelying. The ability of the pelvis and lower extremities to initiate movement and participate in postural activity allows the baby to move the center of gravity over the hip while pushing on the arms. The underside pelvis and femur actively pushes against the floor while the top leg abducts and externally rotates.

The baby is able to move more easily and efficiently between sitting and quadruped through a variety of patterns. In sitting the baby initiates the weight shift by rotating the pelvis over the femur. The trunk rotates from the upper lumbar/lower thoracic area upward as the baby places the hands in a position for weight bearing (figure 7.20). The pelvis then rotates to realign with the shoulders, and the hip can remain adducted as the knee comes into the weight-bearing position. The baby has

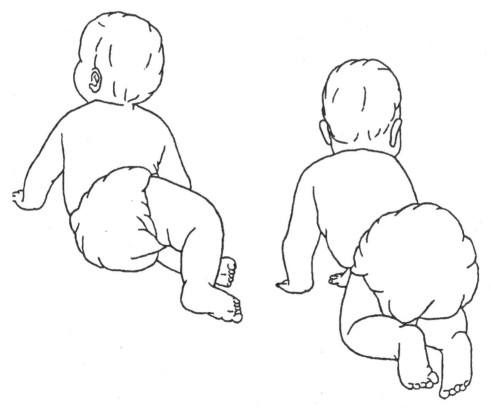

FIGURE 7.20

the option to place the foot on the floor and push in the transition to quadruped. The baby can also initiate the weight shift by moving the pelvis forward over the femurs without arm support (figure 7.21). The arms extend to accept the weight as the center of gravity moves forward.

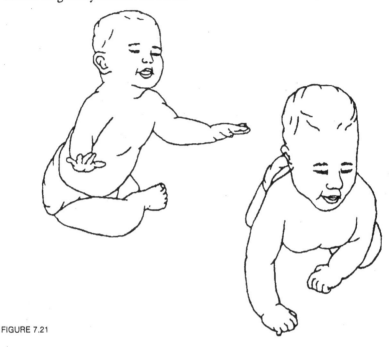

FIGURE 7.21

Transitions from quadruped to sit also demonstrate greater pelvic control and rotation. Rather than a lateral weight shift, the pelvis rotates forward over one knee. The motion occurs at the weight-bearing hip joint; therefore, the pelvis is moving over a fixed femur (external rotation of the hip). The backward rotation of the opposite side of the pelvis unweights that hip, but the foot may provide distal stability by pushing against the floor.

The baby becomes versatile in using a variety of patterns to transition. Rotating from quadruped to sitting results in the baby facing perpendicular to the original position. To accommodate different situations, the baby learns alternate ways to sit up to be more able to orientate the body toward an object (figure 7.22). For example, the baby can face the same direction by placing one foot on the floor and pushing the leg straight while shifting much of the weight to the arms. The baby flexes the unweighted leg forward with abduction and external rotation and lowers the pelvis to sit. This requires considerable proximal stability and the ability to isolate movement of one leg while weight bearing on the other three extremities.

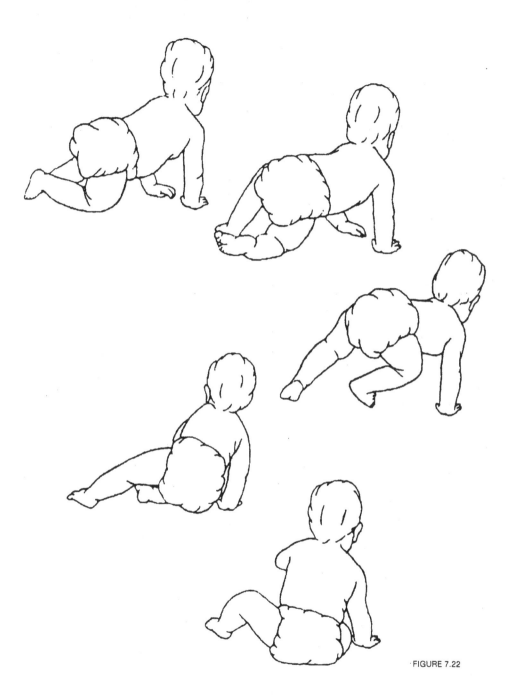

FIGURE 7.22

Quadruped. Postural control continues to develop so that by 12 months of age the child reaches with diagonal trunk control in quadruped. As abdominal and spinal muscle activity hold the trunk elongated, the child reaches one arm forward and extends the opposite leg as a postural accompaniment (figure 7.23).

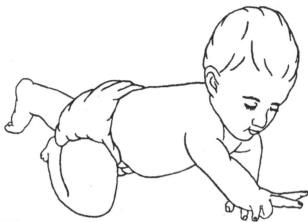

FIGURE 7.23

Increased diagonal postural control allows the child to creep with greater separation (flexion and extension) of the lower extremities. The 10- to 12-month-old child creeps faster and easier than the 8- or 9-month-old child and can push a wheeled toy while creeping. By 12 months old, the child uses trunk rotation to shift the body weight from one set of extremities to the other rather than a purely lateral weight shift (figure 7.24).

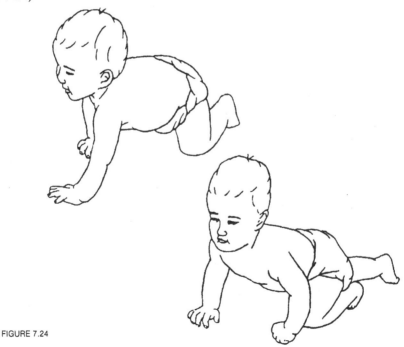

FIGURE 7.24

The 10- to 12-month-old child crawls up stairs; however, on standing upright, the child is in danger of toppling over. The child can turn around and climb backwards off furniture and can be taught to use this pattern to crawl down stairs.

Pulling to standing. The 10- to 12-month-old child uses the lower extremities more actively when pulling up to standing at a support. Shifting the weight laterally in kneeling, the child flexes the nonweight-bearing hip and places the foot on the floor in a half-kneel position (figure 7.25). In contrast to previous months, the child can shift the weight forward to the arms and foot and push against the floor while rising. The opposite leg passively extends until only the foot is touching the floor. The child then flexes the hip and knee to align the foot under the pelvis and adjusts the center of gravity for the desired standing activity. The pattern is not always well coordinated and sometimes the child does not shift the weight quite far enough but still manages to drag the other foot forward.

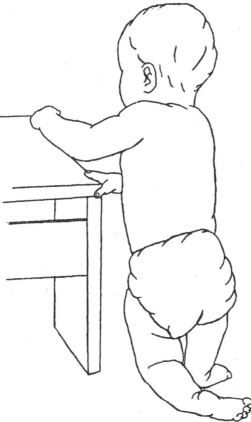

FIGURE 7.25

With repetition, the baby is better able to coordinate postural control with the movement of rising to standing. In stabilizing the posture and controlling the displacement of the center of gravity, the baby requires less support of the arms. By 12 months of age, the baby is able to stand up, using one hand for minimal support, and pull up to less stable surfaces.

The baby also uses the pelvic girdle and lower extremities more actively to stand up from sitting (figure 7.26). The baby can now rotate up over one knee and bring the other foot forward. Shifting the weight to her arms and foot, the baby steps through with the unweighted leg.

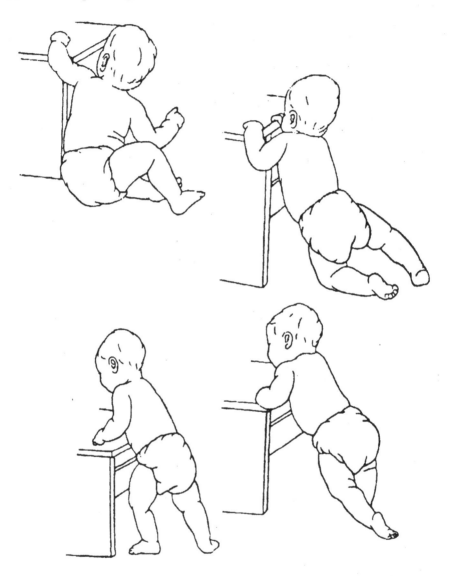

FIGURE 7.26

The 10- to 12-month-old child is able to get down from standing more efficiently. As the child squats, the descent of the center of gravity is controlled by the pelvic/hip/ lower extremity musculature. In particular, the quadriceps contracts eccentrically (as it lengthens) to counteract gravity and grade knee flexion. The child practices squatting over and over, often deliberately dropping toys in order to reach down for them. Initially the child needs the support of both arms to lower the body. As the child develops more control, only one hand is used (figure 7.27). The child may squat to the floor and stand up again, drop the pelvis between the legs and sit, or go forward to quadruped and creep.

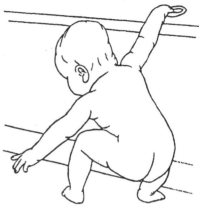

FIGURE 7.27

Standing at furniture becomes more functional because of the baby's increasing ability to free the arms and to control the posture while reaching and playing. However, coordination of posture and movement is just beginning in standing. The baby is not yet able to shift the weight through the pelvis and hips or use subtle postural adjustments to upper body movement. Several strategies provide stability for play. When laterally flexing the trunk to shift the weight sideways, the baby slightly flexes the hips and knees (figure 7.28a). Reaching up or across the body, the baby can support much of the weight on one leg and extend the other back as a postural accompaniment (figure 7.28b). Another strategy involves extending or stiffening of the lower extremities and going up on the toes, either bilaterally or unilaterally (figure 7.28c).

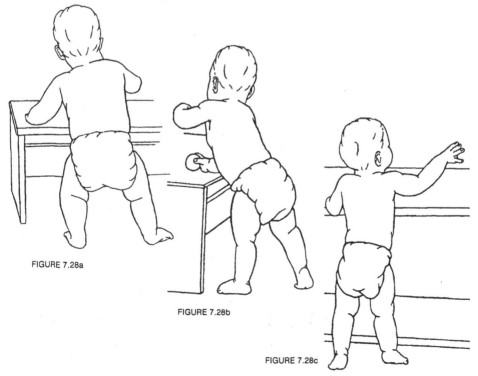

FIGURE 7.28a

FIGURE 7.28b

FIGURE 7.28c

As greater stability develops in standing, the baby begins to move away from the supporting surface. The baby turns diagonally and supports the body with one hand, using the other for function (figure 7.29). The pelvis rotates over the weight-bearing leg with the hips in some degree of flexion, and the trunk is very active, as seen by abdominal activity. The baby is also able to rotate the head and shoulders backward over the supporting leg while holding toys in the hands (figure 7.30).

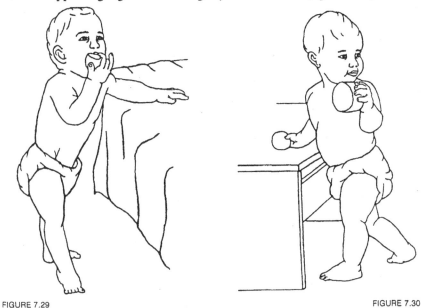

FIGURE 7.29   FIGURE 7.30

Some babies not only turn sideways to the support, but continue to step and turn around so they can lean their buttocks back against the furniture (figure 7.31). Both hands are then free for midline play. Pushing up on the toes provides additional stability.

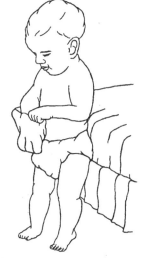

FIGURE 7.31

Many babies seem to have an insatiable desire to stand at this age (Caplan 1971). The child may refuse to lie down, and frustrated parents can become adept at dressing a standing child. Fortunately the child has sufficient balance to hold on to the adult's shoulders and lift one leg for pants, socks, and shoes. Some babies have difficulty sitting long enough for a meal, so finger foods become an important part of their diet for a time. Safety is crucial as, if not properly secured, the baby stands up in the highchair, stroller, or grocery cart.

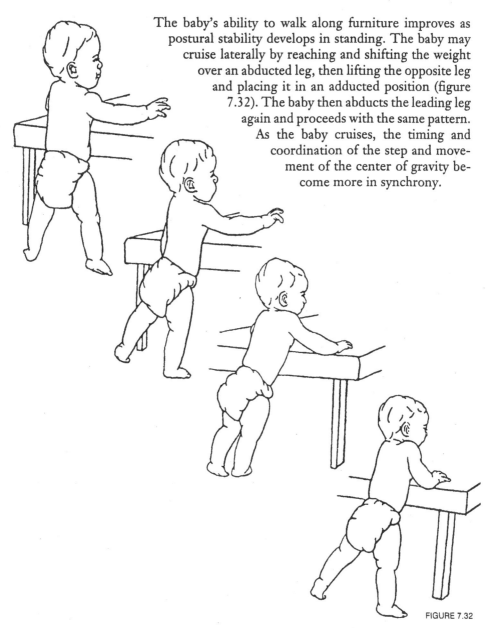

The baby's ability to walk along furniture improves as postural stability develops in standing. The baby may cruise laterally by reaching and shifting the weight over an abducted leg, then lifting the opposite leg and placing it in an adducted position (figure 7.32). The baby then abducts the leading leg again and proceeds with the same pattern. As the baby cruises, the timing and coordination of the step and movement of the center of gravity become more in synchrony.

FIGURE 7.32

The baby may also turn sideways to the support and use a forward stepping movement to cruise (figure 7.33). The pattern appears to be well coordinated and a heel-toe gait pattern may be seen in some babies. This is a more efficient pattern because the baby does not have to shift the center of gravity laterally from one leg to the other while stepping. However, the baby needs to control forward movement of the body mass. At times the trunk may lag behind the legs in stepping, but at other times the baby is able to move it along with the forward movement of the legs.

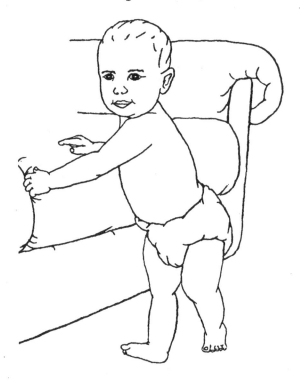

FIGURE 7.33

There appear to be many individual differences in babies' desires to cruise and the patterns they use. Some babies who are floppy or heavier take longer to develop standing control and may never use cruising; rather they go right to independent walking when their systems are ready. Others use a variety of patterns, turning diagonally or sideways to the support. Some take only a step or two to get to an object and others seem driven to walk from one piece of furniture to the next. Many babies cruise only in a familiar environment along a favorite support such as the living room sofa. Others pull up to standing and walk along or around any stable surface.

In addition to cruising, the baby may discover that by pushing a kitchen-type chair, the chair moves. The baby then takes a step toward it, pushes, and it moves again. Soon the baby is pushing the chair around the room. Sturdy, wheeled toys are now commercially available that provide sufficient stability for a baby who is not yet walking independently.

The baby may also enjoy walking with one hand held (figure 7.34). The free arm raises in abduction and the hand opens as a postural accompaniment to stabilize the upper body. In stepping, the baby begins to shift the weight laterally over the supporting leg. Initially the baby loses control, pivots around the leg on the supported side, and collapses or hangs from the arm. With repetition the baby learns to control and alternate the weight shift in preparation for independent walking.

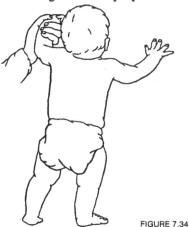

FIGURE 7.34

Independent standing and walking. By 11 and 12 months, most babies have sufficient coordination of posture and movement to stand at a variety of supports that provide less stability. This is an important phase in the progression to independent standing and walking. While learning more proximal postural control, grasp and toe flexion are used as a form of distal stability. For example, an adult's shirt offers a flexible support that gives variable amounts of tension as it is pulled (7.35a). A plastic laundry basket or cardboard box used to hold toys provides another flexible support (7.35b). The oral mechanism may also contribute to distal stability as seen in this baby's tongue (7.35c). Babies learn to squat, reach, and play using less stable supports just as they once learned to use furniture.

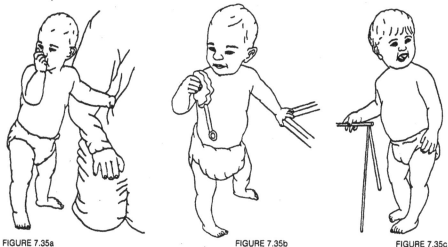

FIGURE 7.35a   FIGURE 7.35b   FIGURE 7.35c

As postural control develops, while standing with minimal support of one hand, the baby releases the grasp and keeps only minimal contact (figure 7.36). If motivated to use that hand, the baby may let go and the entire body sets itself to be stable. The hips, knees, and toes flex while the opposite arm assumes a similar pattern to the interactive arm. Symmetry provides stability, whereas asymmetry is posturally destabilizing. When babies realize they are standing alone, their arms spread out, their hips flex, and they fall to sitting.

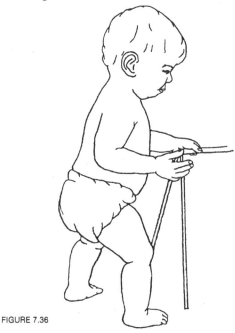

FIGURE 7.36

Often the first independent standing occurs accidentally when the baby is walking from one supporting surface to another. The baby takes a step, stops, and reaches for the next support with one hand while letting go with the other. Some babies begin to take two or three steps before using an arm for support again. In this way they gradually begin to walk independently. It may take several weeks or months for them to feel secure and walk longer distances.

In contrast to babies who stand alone briefly and take a step, other babies begin to take steps before they demonstrate independent standing. Seemingly driven to walk, they take off across the room, falling from foot to foot until they lose their balance or run into furniture. They are unable to coordinate the movement with their emerging postural control.

The first conscious independent steps may require all the child's efforts and concentration. As one parent lets go, the child focuses the eyes on the other parent, abducts the arms and stiffly takes a few steps until caught (Caplan 1971). Motivation is enhanced by the smiling faces and applause received from the parents, and repeating the game is an important part of learning to walk.

About the time of learning to walk independently, the baby also begins to stand up from the floor without support. From quadruped the baby pushes up on the hands and feet, then shifts the center of gravity back, and lowers the pelvis to a squat position. Lifting the head and upper trunk, the baby pushes the feet against the floor and extends the knees and hips until upright (figure 7.37). The baby also learns to stand up from sitting by moving into a squat (figure 7.38). With one foot on the floor, the baby leans forward on the arms while lifting the pelvis and places the other foot on the floor. The baby then shifts the weight back over the feet and rises to standing. As postural control continues to develop in standing, the baby also begins to squat to play (figure 7.39). Soon the baby is walking, squatting, then walking again.

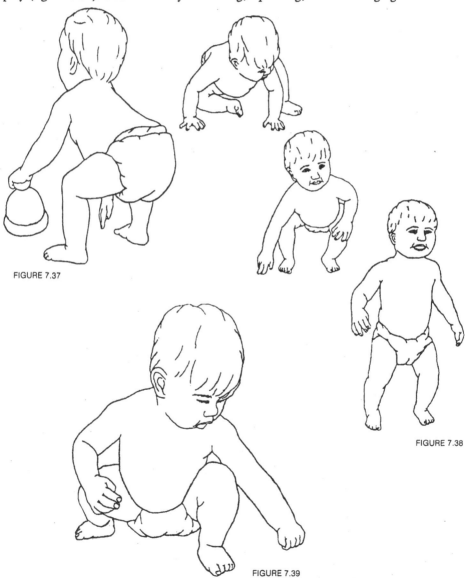

FIGURE 7.37

FIGURE 7.38

FIGURE 7.39

Initially, babies take off toward a target, but may find themselves going in a different direction because walking in a straight line is difficult. Babies cannot always make the corrections needed, so their attention easily shifts to another target. When they first start walking independently, babies cannot stop or turn around without support. As they learn to control the momentum of walking, they stop and take small circular steps to turn, but balance is precarious and they use posturing of the arms for additional stability.

The age at which a child begins to walk is extremely variable, with some babies walking as early as 9 months of age and others not until 16 months. The average age for independent walking in the United States is 12 to 14 months (Caplan 1971). When ready to walk, the baby rather quickly develops the coordination of posture and movement needed for function. In a matter of weeks, the baby walks to objects, squats, and picks them up. Pull toys and push toys give enjoyment as the baby practices this new skill. Walking to cupboards or drawers, the baby quickly learns to open and close them. The ability to stand and walk creates a new and expanded environment that affects all areas of development.

Gait. Current theory suggests that the movement patterns for walking are generated by a central program of neural control (Myklebust 1990). The basic pattern can be elicited during the newborn period and is referred to as automatic stepping. The program is modified as maturation and motor learning occur, particularly to include the postural control necessary for balance. Morphological changes such as body weight also have an impact. The beginning walker demonstrates patterns that reflect the immature level of postural control. By 18 months of age, postural activity is fairly well coordinated with walking and the baby uses a pattern similar to mature gait. The variables that determine further maturity are related to the musculoskeletal system (for example, limb length) was well as to stability (Sutherland et al. 1980).

Throughout the gait cycle, the toddler uses certain patterns to provide the stability necessary for independent walking. The hips are flexed and externally rotated and the feet are apart for a wide base of support (figure 7.40a). The spine is extended in the thoraco-lumbar area and extends more to control the forward displacement of body mass that results from momentum (figures 7.40b, c, d). The elbows flex to control the distal part of the arm and help stabilize the shoulder girdle and upper trunk. The arms abduct if more stability is needed (see figure 7.40b). Rotation of the humerus varies according to the destabilizing forces acting on the upper body. External rotation often occurs when the force is directed anteriorly and accompanies increased spinal extension to keep the center of gravity more posterior (see figures 7.40c, d). The oral mechanism contributes to stability of the head, neck, and shoulders.

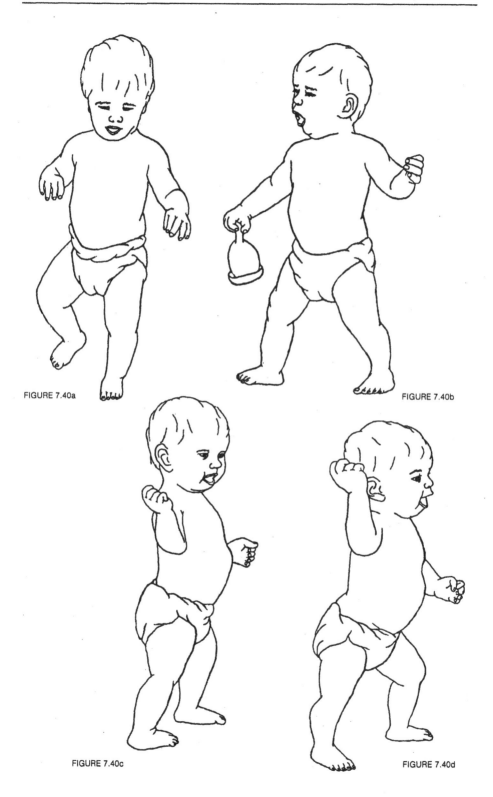

FIGURE 7.40a

FIGURE 7.40b

FIGURE 7.40c

FIGURE 7.40d

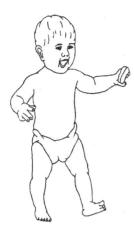

During the swing phase of gait, hip and knee flexion is greater in early walking patterns and the limb is propelled forward by rotation of the pelvis and hip as well as lumbar extension (anterior tilt of the pelvis). During the latter part of the swing phase, the baby may hold the foot dorsiflexed while extending the knee, similar to the more mature heel-toe pattern (figure 7.41). However, the ankle begins to plantar flex just before it touches the ground so the initial contact is made by the ball of the foot. This may reflect not only insufficient control of the dorsiflexion, but lack of controlled lateral and rotational pelvic movement to lower the limb to the floor. The plantar flexion also provides stability to the ankle in preparation for weight bearing.

FIGURE 7.41

EMG studies reveal cocontraction of the muscles anterior and posterior to the ankle (anterior tibialis and gastrocnemius) during the stance phase (Berger et al. 1984). This begins to decrease at about two years of age and a reciprocal innervation pattern appears in which the anterior tibialis becomes silent during stance. The early pattern provides greater ankle stability for maintaining postural control.

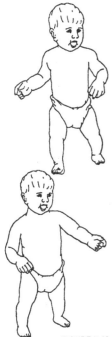

In order to step, the body weight must be transferred to one leg. The toddler shifts the weight through a lateral displacement of the head, shoulder, and upper body (figure 7.42) and quickly steps with the free leg, lifting it high in the air. The toddler then moves the head and shoulders to that side and takes a step with the trailing leg. Learning to coordinate the weight shift with movement is difficult and the baby often appears to be out of control. The timing of steps is not always rhythmical. Sometimes the baby momentarily stops with the weight on one leg, wobbles, and tries to keep balanced. Postural reactions may be seen if the baby shifts the weight too far laterally. The arms abduct and a righting reaction is seen in the trunk that may bring the center of gravity under control. Since postural reactions are controlled by a feedback mechanism, the reaction may happen too late and the baby falls. As postural accompaniments develop and are coordinated with the walking pattern, the baby loses balance less frequently and stepping becomes more rhythmical.

As the baby develops stability in walking, less posturing of the arms is seen. Initially one or both arms are flexed at the elbows and in various amounts of abduction. As the baby walks, the

FIGURE 7.42

arms move in and out of the more stabilizing positions. One arm may relax at the side, only to spring up again as the baby takes an unsteady step or makes a turn. It will be several months before the baby is able to walk with the arms free from this type of postural activity. A reciprocal arm swing emerges around 18 months of age.

■ Fine Motor Development

This is an exciting period of time for children as they develop proficiency in the way they use their hands in play and during self-care. They may not always be graceful, but through successive approximation, they experiment with toys and imitate the adult's use of tools (Caplan 1971). They know what they want to do and use trial and error to independently achieve their objectives. For example, when not able to reach the cookie on the table, the baby may simply pull on the tablecloth or pull the table over to get what is wanted. This is a good time for parents to put away their breakable mementos, because the reach of the 10- to 12-month old child is accurate and quick. The child attempts to hold as many objects as possible and explores anything within reach.

Hand Development

From 10 to 12 months of age, the child may demonstrate a hand preference. This is reflected in the new way the child holds an object with one hand and manipulates it with the preferred hand (figure 7.43). The child may also hold a container with one hand and attempt to remove the lid with the preferred hand. This is the beginning of bimanual hand development wherein each hand has a different motor task within the same function. Bimanual dexterity is the prerequisite for cutting food and using scissors, skills acquired in later years.

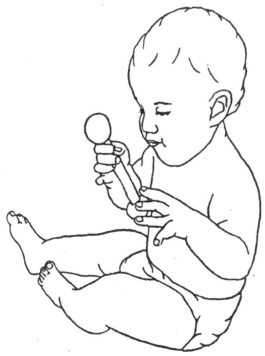

FIGURE 7.43

The child enjoys manipulating objects with two hands by pushing, pulling, squeezing, and rotating (figures 7.44a, b, and c). The child delights in putting objects in containers and may tip over the container to obtain the toys. Blocks are enjoyable, and the child may attempt to stack two of them, usually without being successful (figure 7.45). The child is attracted to toys with moveable parts and observable actions (figure 7.46). The child turns the pages of a book, although not necessarily one at a time, and enjoys looking at the pictures (figure 7.47). Because of increased dexterity, children at this age can amuse themselves for longer periods. For example, the child may remove a sock, put it someplace, and never show you where it is. The child is now eagerly combining many different fine motor patterns into function.

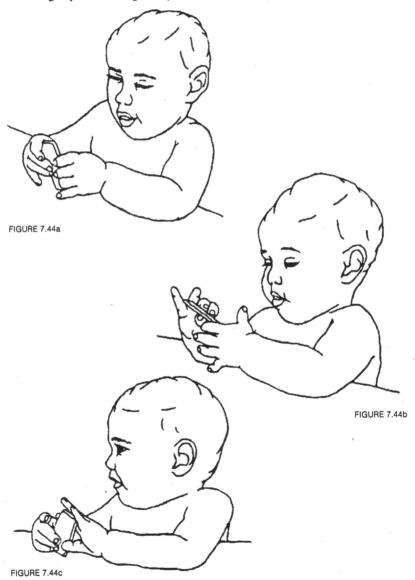

FIGURE 7.44a

FIGURE 7.44b

FIGURE 7.44c

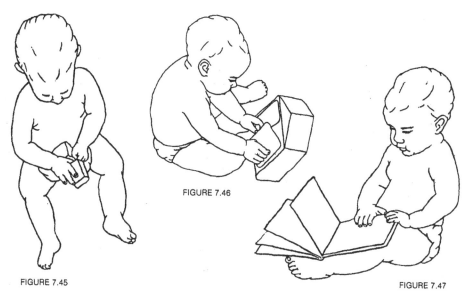

FIGURE 7.46

FIGURE 7.45

FIGURE 7.47

The child at this age has mastered the three-jaw chuck, but finds this prehension insufficient for pellet-sized objects (figure 7.48). The 10-month-old baby discovers the pincer grasp where small objects such as dry cereal are obtained between the distal pads of the thumb and index finger (figure 7.49). By 12 months of age, the baby can pinch, using the tips of the finger and thumb, eventually gaining greater thumb rotation with practice (figure 7.50). Equipped with this new skill, children are capable of retrieving and swallowing coins, safety pins, and other small objects hidden in the carpet, between cushions, or under furniture.

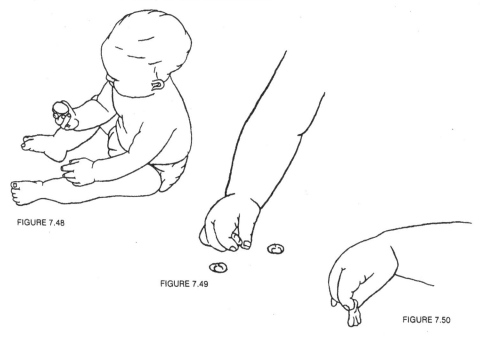

FIGURE 7.48

FIGURE 7.49

FIGURE 7.50

The 10- to 12-month-old child fingerfeeds with more proficiency. The extent of the child's "table manners" is related to both oral and fine motor control. This complicated motor task, when done gracefully, combines intricate patterns of motion between the elbow, forearm, wrist, and hand to orient finger foods toward and into the mouth (figure 7.51). The child has a finer sense of pressure on delicate foods such as crackers. However, some children are less adept than others (figures 7.52a, b, c, d).

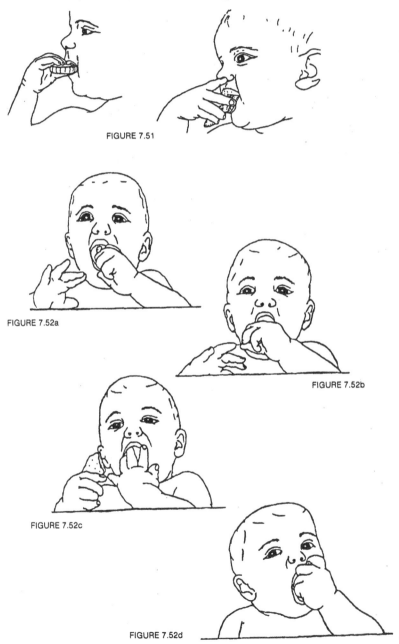

FIGURE 7.51

FIGURE 7.52a

FIGURE 7.52b

FIGURE 7.52c

FIGURE 7.52d

At this age, babies may cupdrink independently with consistent spilling. They attempt to spoonfeed themselves, but are usually unsuccessful at using this important tool (figure 7.53). Through imitation babies learn about the specific use of tools for their intended purpose. They put a comb to the head and a toothbrush in the mouth, but do not yet have the motor control to orient the tool properly for the task.

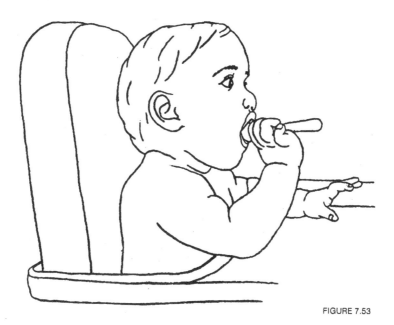

FIGURE 7.53

At 12 months of age, the child has the full body control for beginning independence in the world. The child's fine motor skills will continue to develop over time, leading toward greater and greater levels of creativity, discovery, and autonomy.

■ Oral-Motor and Respiratory Development

Anatomical/Structural Characteristics

The oral and pharyngeal mechanisms. The oral and pharyngeal mechanisms of babies 10 to 12 months old are significantly different in the contour, shape, size, and alignment of their structures and musculature when compared to their oral and pharyngeal mechanisms as newborn infants. Growth, nutrition, and the development of coordinated musculature activity through movement have already dramatically changed these mechanisms. However, the baby's oral and pharyngeal mechanisms still have many more changes to undergo before reaching adult structural alignment and function.

The oral cavity, nasopharynx, oropharynx, and laryngopharynx of the adult (figure 7.54) are significantly different from those of a newborn infant and a 12-month-old child. (See figures 2.13, 2.14, and 2.15 in Chapter 2 for a comparison.) Not only are the mouth and pharynx of the adult larger and more elongated, but also the alignment of their structures suggests the dependence of the adult on well-controlled musculature activity to coordinate intricate functional movements of the structures of the mechanisms for eating, swallowing, respiratory, and speech activities. The structures, alignment, and functional abilities of the oral and pharyngeal mechanisms of the 12-month-old baby will continue to modify as described in Chapter 4 through puberty until adult structure and function are achieved.

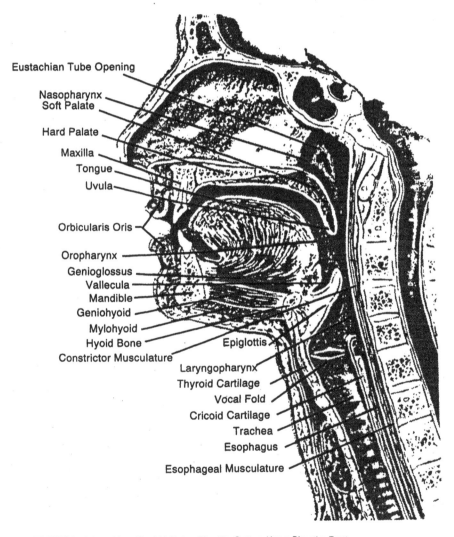

FIGURE 7.54. Adapted from Frank H. Netter, Digestive System: Upper Digestive Tract from *CIBA Collection of Medical Illustrations* (West Caldwell, NJ: CIBA Pharmaceutical Co., 1959), section 1 (plate 16).

Rib cage and diaphragm. As the abdominal and shoulder girdle musculature provide active sources of stability for the downwardly-rotated rib cage, and as the intercostal muscles between the ribs elongate and become more active, increased rib cage mobility is evident as the 10- to 12-month-old child experiences a greater variety of movement activities. Changes in the contour and shape of the rib cage are evident as the infant uses more coordinated musculature activity to move from sitting to quadruped (figure 7.55), creep on hands and knees (figure 7.56), side sit (figure 7.57), stand (figure 7.58), and move up to and down from standing (figure 7.59). The structures and musculature of the rib cage are now free to actively assist the baby to control movements through wider ranges of weightshift and to establish a more active base of postural control through the trunk.

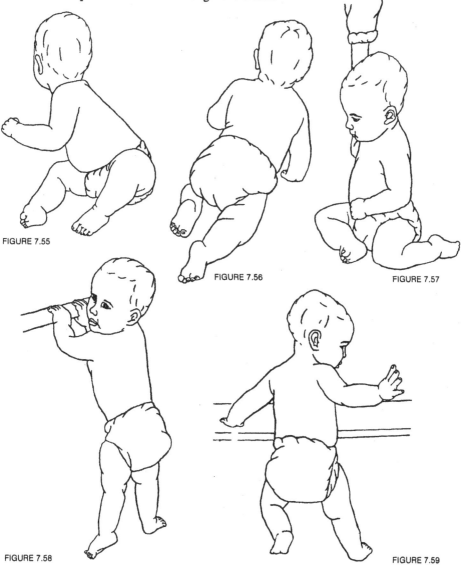

FIGURE 7.55

FIGURE 7.56

FIGURE 7.57

FIGURE 7.58

FIGURE 7.59

The intercostal muscles are becoming more active during the respiratory process. Therefore, lateral and anterior-posterior expansion of the rib cage is seen more often in coordination with more efficient diaphragm activity on inhalation. This results in increased air intake in conjunction with decreasing respiratory rates.

By 12 months of age, the nonrespiratory structures, or conducting airways, of the lungs (trachea, bronchi, and bronchioles) are increasing in their lengths and diameters. The number and size of respiratory structures within the lungs have also shown major change, resulting in a significantly increased total lung volume (Green and Doershuk 1985).

The baby gradually develops a more adult abdominal-thoracic breathing pattern over the next few years as the muscles of inhalation (diaphragm, external and internal intercostals, levatores costarum, serratus posterior superior, latissimus dorsi, sternocleidomastoid, scaleni anterior, medius, and posterior, subclavius, pectoralis major and minor, serratus anterior) and the muscles of exhalation (transversus thoracis, internal intercostals, subcostal muscles, serratus posterior inferior, quadratus lumborum, external and internal obliques, transversus abdominus, rectus abdominus) develop more active, coordinated functional activity. The shape and contour of the rib cage continue to modify through puberty with growth and greater expansion and elongation of the chest wall. (See figures 2.7 and 2.8 in Chapter 2.)

Developmental Characteristics

Babies from 10 to 12 months of age are learning to coordinate oral-motor activity with the wide variety of gross motor and fine motor activities they are involved in throughout the day. They experiment with up, down, and lateral-diagonal movements of the jaw; up-down, forward-backward, and lateral movements of the tongue; and closure, rounding, and spreading (retraction) of the lips in sitting (figures 7.60 and 7.61), in standing (figure 7.62), and when creeping on hands and knees (figure 7.63). Babies often make sounds and engage in feeding and drinking activities as they learn to coordinate respiratory, pharyngeal, and oral function (figure 7.64). As they play with their oral movements in various body positions and gross motor activities, they discover new ways to functionally control and coordinate movements of the jaw, tongue, and lips. Drooling rarely occurs, but when it does, it usually relates to teething.

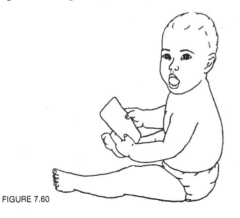

FIGURE 7.60

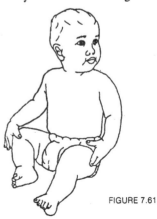

FIGURE 7.61

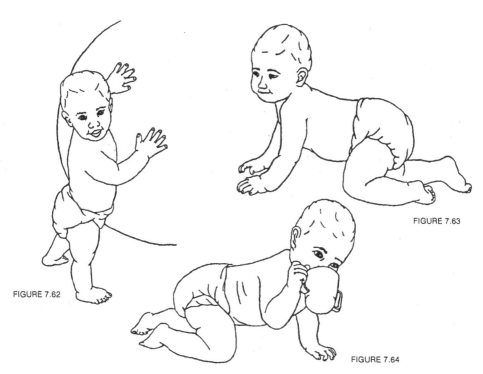

FIGURE 7.63

FIGURE 7.62

FIGURE 7.64

Limited oral activity and greater posturing of the oral mechanism for distal stability are evident when infants independently pull up to standing at less stable support surfaces (figure 7.65), when they begin to take their first independent steps, and when they are enthusiastically focused on new upper extremity activities. Drooling occurs during these activities, gradually decreasing as babies develop greater control of their movements and learn to coordinate oral activity more effectively with them.

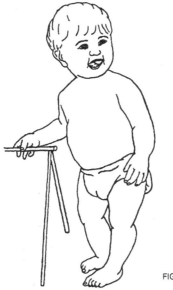

FIGURE 7.65

The feeding process. Infants between 10 and 12 months of age are placed in a highchair at a 90-degree angle for feeding without any external supports necessary. Seat belts and trays need to be used for safety reasons because babies at this age often like to stand up and climb out of the highchair. By 18 to 24 months of age, the child may be introduced to a booster seat or junior chair that can be brought up to the family table at mealtime. Although the highchair may continue to be used, it is not required for assuring the child's safety and security.

From 10 to 12 months, the baby is increasing liquid intake from the cup, while decreasing the need for liquid intake by bottledrinking and breastfeeding. Parents often begin transitioning the baby to cupdrinking gradually by reducing the number of bottles or time spent breastfeeding during the day. Many children continue to bottledrink or breastfeed before naps or at bedtimes until approximately two years of age. This relates most directly to their use of oral sucking activity for calming and quieting rather than their need for liquid intake at these times.

A more mature sucking pattern of the oral mechanism is emerging from 10 to 12 months with more coordinated, short sequences of sucking and swallowing in cupdrinking (figure 7.66). Forward and backward movements of the tongue are observed less often even as the cup is presented or removed. Liquid loss greatly reduces, but does still occur.

Although the oral-motor activity of the child during cupdrinking is significantly more organized and coordinated, up/down and forward/backward movements of the jaw in wide excursions continue to occur (figure 7.67). To compensate for this jaw instability, some babies protrude the tongue slightly under the cup and bring the

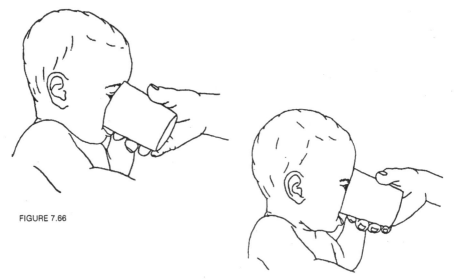

FIGURE 7.66

FIGURE 7.67

lower lip up to surround the tongue, creating a more stable foundation for oral activity (figures 7.68a and b). The upper lip is postured downward, but may not yet actively close on the cup rim. Some 12-month-old children maintain the tongue within the oral mechanism during sucking, but alternate between intermittent tongue tip elevation and tongue protrusion when swallowing.

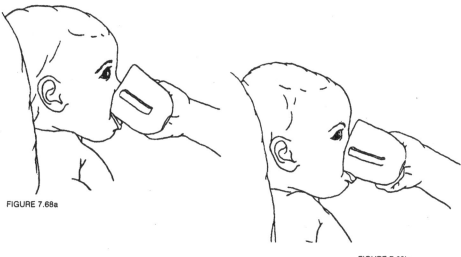

FIGURE 7.68a

FIGURE 7.68b

Oral-motor activity in coordination with swallowing and breathing during cup drinking will continue to develop gradually over the next year. Between 12 and 15 months of age many children begin biting on the cup rim for jaw stability, while obtaining active closure of the upper and lower lips and active controlled movements of the tongue to guide the liquid back for well coordinated sucking and swallowing (Morris 1982). By 24 months of age, the child holds the cup rim between the lips as internal jaw stabilization and more consistent tongue elevation on swallowing emerge. Children continue to use a mixture of oral and pharyngeal movement patterns after 24 months until a more adult system for handling liquids by cup is achieved.

The textures of foods handled by babies from 10 to 12 months of age is gradually changing to include coarsely chopped table foods. By 12 months, babies may also be getting soft cooked chicken and ground meats to eat. Toddlers 18 to 24 months of age are eating a wider variety of chopped foods such as meats and raw vegetables. They exhibit definite preferences for certain foods as they begin to exert their independence about which foods they wish to eat or not eat at a meal. This can create some major frustrations for parents at mealtime.

At 10 months of age, as the spoon is presented, the baby actively moves the body forward over the hips, lowers the jaw, keeps the tongue quiet within the mouth, and brings the lips forward. Once the spoon enters the mouth, the baby moves the lower lip up to hold under the spoon while the upper lip moves downward (figure 7.69). As the spoon is being drawn out, the upper lip moves inward to remove the food from the spoon and the lower lip moves inward until the spoon is removed and lip closure is achieved. Babies use head flexion to assist as they close their lips on the spoon for food removal (figure 7.70). As they are able to initiate a controlled weight shift backward while sitting in the highchair, they also begin to use this movement with lip closure as part of the spoonfeeding process (figure 7.71).

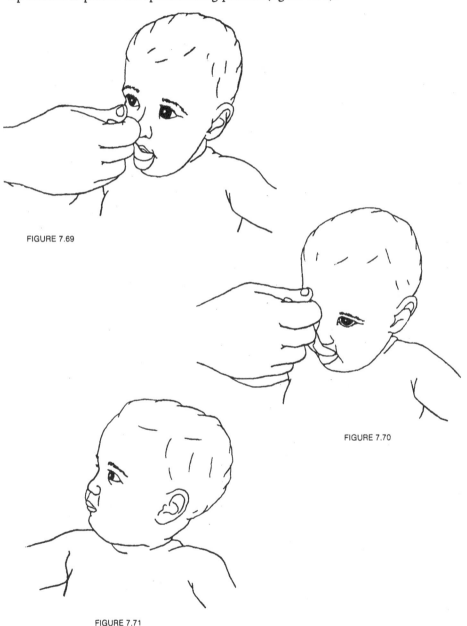

FIGURE 7.69

FIGURE 7.70

FIGURE 7.71

By 12 months of age, this process for removing food from a spoon is well organized. Any food remaining on the lower lip is removed as the lower lip draws inward so food can be scraped off by the upper teeth. By 24 months, the child uses the tongue to clean food from the upper and lower lips.

Up-and-down movements of the tongue and jaw characteristic of sucking are emerging as suckling movements decrease during spoonfeeding from 10 to 12 months of age. Easy tongue protrusion is used during swallowing, although intermittent elevation of the front of the tongue may also be evident. Over the next year, children develop more precise up/down movements of the tongue for handling semisolids in the mouth and more consistent tongue tip elevation for swallowing. Although more adult-like movements of the oral mechanism are used by the 24-month-old during spoonfeeding, further refinement of tongue activity occurs through the third year (Morris and Klein 1987).

The 10- to 12-month-old baby is developing a more controlled, sustained bite through a soft solid such as a soft cookie or cracker (figure 7.72). The baby generally places the cookie or cracker in the front of the mouth between the central incisors, elevates the jaw to close on the cookie, gradually bites through the cookie, and releases the bite easily for chewing (figure 7.73). Although the baby's lips often close on the soft cookie during the biting process, lip closure is not always used.

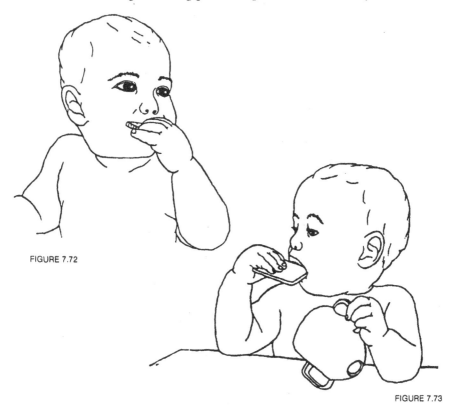

FIGURE 7.72

FIGURE 7.73

The 12-month-old child who has both upper and lower central incisors may use a controlled, sustained bite through a hard solid. If the strength of the bite is not yet powerful enough, the child may close the jaw to hold on the hard solid before breaking a piece off with the hands. Phasic up/down jaw movements and sucking activity may also be used on the hard solid. By 24 months of age, the child uses a controlled, sustained bite through soft and hard solids, grading the size of the jaw opening needed to bite through a variety of food thicknesses.

Jaw and tongue movements used during chewing from 10 to 12 months of age are similar to those seen at 9 months. The baby is gaining more experience in transferring food from the center to the sides of the mouth, using lateral movements of the tongue, and in breaking up the food on the side, using diagonal rotary movements of the jaw (figure 7.74). By 12 months the baby is transferring food from the center to both sides of the mouth with tongue lateralization, although the baby often needs to pause in the center when moving food from one side to the other. Forward and backward movements of the tongue may be used intermittently when food is in the center of the mouth. Up-and-down jaw movements also may occur.

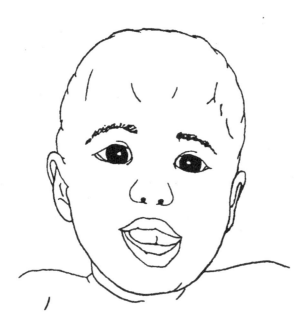

FIGURE 7.74

The cheeks and lips become significantly more active during chewing in the 10- to 12-month period. The lower lip draws inward so the upper teeth or gums can be used to clean food off (figure 7.75). As the baby chews food on the side of the mouth, the cheek and lip musculature on that side may begin to tighten slightly and draw inward. This newly emerging activity of the cheeks and corners of the lips coordinates with the lateral movements of the tongue to keep food on the biting surfaces for chewing. Although the lips are more active during the chewing process, food and saliva may still be lost. Intermittently elevated anterior tongue activity alternates with simple tongue protrusion during swallowing (figure 7.76).

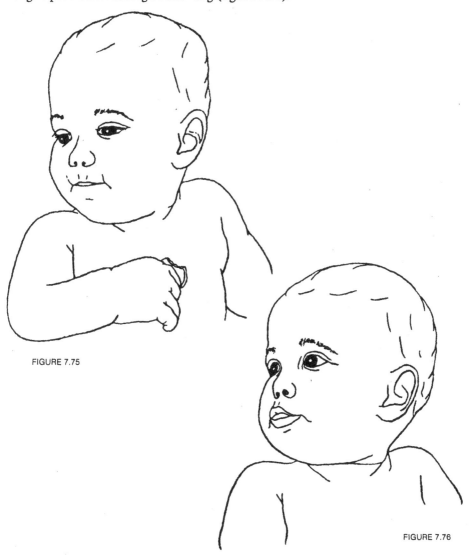

FIGURE 7.75

FIGURE 7.76

During the next year, children learn to coordinate activity of the tongue, jaw, lips, and cheeks more effectively for chewing. Side-to-side tongue movements and diagonal rotary jaw movements gradually become more organized. Lip closure is used more frequently. As the tongue moves food from one side of the mouth to the other in a smoother manner, circular rotary movements of the jaw begin to emerge at approximately 24 months of age (Morris and Klein 1987).

Children and adults use a variety of oral-motor patterns during chewing. The texture, size, and shape of the solids are all factors that directly influence the jaw, tongue, and lip activity used and the amount of time needed to bite through and chew different foods (Archambault et al. 1990; Gisel 1991). As the oral mechanism modifies with growth and the child is introduced to a wider variety of food experiences, a well-coordinated mixture of oral movements for chewing will gradually develop through three to four years of age.

Significant components of respiratory function. Belly breathing with belly expansion on inhalation continues to be the primary respiratory pattern for 10- to 12-month-old babies. When crying or involved in activities that allow the abdominal obliques to more effectively stabilize the lower rib cage, thoracic expansion characteristic of an abdominal-thoracic breathing pattern occurs. As babies continue to develop greater postural control, abdominal musculature activity and strength, and greater activity of the intercostals, the occurrence of thoracic expansion on inhalation increases and the chest appears more rectangular in shape. Abdominal-thoracic breathing continues to develop over the next year, modifying in its structural and physiological foundations during puberty with further growth of the trunk and maturation of the pulmonary system.

With greater expansion of the thoracic area and more effective and efficient diaphragm activity, the baby's air intake is increasing while the respiratory rates are decreasing. At 12 months of age, respiratory rates are more adult-like. The baby's respiratory rate during crying now approximates the adult's range of respiratory rates for speech. Changes in the baby's respiratory pattern, musculature control of inhalation and exhalation coordination, and rate of respiration suggest that the respiratory foundation will soon be prepared for speech production (Redstone 1991).

From 10 to 12 months of age, babies play with more controlled movement of their oral mechanisms on a more actively stable postural base (figure 7.77). They begin producing long chains of sounds composed of different consonant-vowel combinations (variegated or non-reduplicated babbling). Finer oral-motor control is used to create new fricative sounds (for example, /f/, /v/, /s/, /z/) in combination with vowels. New vowel productions are made as the shape and contour of the oral mechanism is changing the resonating cavity and as the tongue, jaw, and lips exhibit new and more coordinated movements. From 12 months on, children begin to produce their first real words and begin to change from babbling to jargon with more adult-like stress and intonation patterns. They are combining many methods of communication (for example, facial expression, pointing, and sound/speech production) as they explore and interact in the world around them.

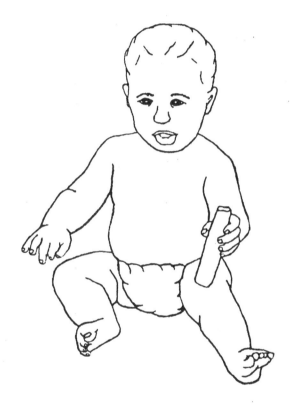

FIGURE 7.77

Summary Chart—10-12 Months

Postural Control	Gross Motor	Fine Motor
Equilibrium reactions refined in sitting and quadruped, beginning in kneeling and standing	Dynamic sitting with greater variety of patterns; improved ability to reach and play	Masters the three-jaw chuck
Protective extension of the arms backwards in sitting (10 months)	Sits on small chair or stool	Pincer grasp with finger and thumb pads at 10 months
Increased postural activity of the pelvic girdle and hips	Sits up from sidelying	Finger-tip pinch developing at 12 months
Efficient postural alignment with "S" spinal curve	More efficient transitions sitting/ quadruped/standing	May develop hand preference
Increased postural activity of lower extremities	Creeps upstairs	Developing bimanual dexterity
Initiates and controls weight shift from the pelvic girdle in sitting and transitions	Lowers self backward off furniture	Manipulates by pushing, pulling, squeezing, and rotating
	Pulls to stand and lowers self using less stable surfaces	Combines fine motor patterns into function
	Stands with less support; improved ability to reach and play	• removes socks and unties shoes • fingerfeeding and cupdrinking skills improve • attempts spoon feeding with minimal success • imitates adult's use of tools, such as combing his hair
	Begins independent standing	
	Stands up without support through squat	
	Walks with one hand held; pushes chair	
	Begins independent walking	

Some infants develop activities earlier or later than this chart indicates. Therefore, it should not be regarded as a rigid timetable of events.

Summary Chart—10-12 Months continued

Oral-Motor/Feeding	Respiration-Phonation
Feeding	*Respiration*
Coordinates long sequences of sucking-swallowing-breathing on bottle/breast; begins to be weaned from bottle with increasing liquid intake by cup (12 months)	Belly breathing with minimal rib flaring most often used
Coordinates short sequences of sucking-swallowing on the cup with less liquid loss	Abdominal-thoracic breathing pattern developing; thoracic expansion occurs during crying and activities when the abdominal obliques are most active
• uses wide up/down and forward/backward jaw movements	
• may protrude tongue and elevate lower lip under cup for stability	*Phonation/Sounds*
• postures upper lip downward	Produces phonation/sounds separate from active body movement
• may use tongue protrusion and intermittent anterior tongue elevation on swallow (12 months)	
Opens/quiets mouth and brings body forward as spoon approaches	Produces long chains of different consonant-vowel combinations (non-reduplicated babbling)
• easily closes lips on spoon	
• moves upper lip inward to clean food off spoon	Begins to produce fricatives in combination with vowels
• moves lower lip inward as spoon is removed and lips close	
• uses head flexion to assist in lip closure on spoon	Begins to produce high front, mid back, and high back vowels
• may shift trunk and head back with lip closure as spoon is removed from mouth (11 to 12 months)	
• scrapes food off lower lip with upper teeth (12 months)	May produce first real words (12 months)
• uses sucking with intermittent suckling to move food back	May begin to use jargon (12 months)
• uses tongue protrusion and intermittent anterior tongue elevation on swallow	
Uses controlled, sustained bite on soft cookie/cracker	
• may posture, hold, and break off piece of hard solid or use phasic up/down jaw movements	
• may use controlled, sustained bite on hard solid if upper and lower teeth are present (12 months)	
Chews with mixture of up/down and diagonal rotary jaw movements	
• moves food center-to-sides with tongue lateralization	
• may move food side-to-side with tongue, but must pause in center (12 months)	
• cleans food off lower lip with teeth	
• cheeks and lip corners draw inward on side with food to help keep food on biting surfaces	
• alternates simple tongue protrusion with intermittent anterior tongue elevation on swallow	
Oral-Motor	
Produces more coordinated jaw, tongue, and lip movement when sitting, standing, and creeping on hands and knees; drooling rarely occurs except when teething	
May posture mouth for stability or produce less oral activity when pulling to stand independently, taking first independent steps, and focused on new upper extremity activities; may drool	

■ References

Archambault, M., K. Millen, and E. Gisel. 1990. Effect of bite size on eating development in normal children 6 months to 2 years of age. *Physical and Occupational Therapy in Pediatrics* 10(4):29-47.

Berger, W., E. Altenmueller, and V. Dietz. 1984. Normal and impaired development of children's gait. *Human Biology* 3:163-70.

Caplan, F. 1971. *The first twelve months of life.* New York: Grosset and Dunlap.

Gisel, E. 1991. Effect of food texture on the development of chewing of children between six months and two years of age. *Developmental Medicine and Child Neurology* 33:69-79.

Green, C. C., and C. F. Doershuk. 1985. Development of the respiratory system. In *Pediatric respiratory therapy*, edited by M. D. Lough, C. F. Doershuk, and R. C. Stern, 1-24. Chicago: Year Book Medical Publishers, Inc.

Morris, S. E. 1982. *The normal acquisition of oral feeding skills: Implications for assessment and treatment.* Santa Barbara, CA: Therapeutic Media.

Morris, S. E., and M. D. Klein. 1987. *Pre-Feeding skills.* Tucson, AZ: Therapy Skill Builders.

Myklebust, B. 1990. A review of myotatic reflexes and the development of motor control and gait in infants and children: A special communication. *Physical Therapy* 70:188-203.

Redstone, F. 1991. Respiratory components of communication. In *Neurodevelopmental strategies for managing communication disorders in children with severe motor dysfunction*, edited by M. B. Langley and L. J. Lombardino, 29-48. Austin, TX: Pro-Ed.

Sutherland, D., R. Olshen, L. Cooper, and S. Woo. 1980. The development of mature gait. *Journal of Bone and Joint Surgery* 62:336-53.

Chapter 8

Speech and Language Development

Ruth Saletsky Kamen, Ph.D.

While learning speech, the child must gain proficiency in both vocalization and articulation. Oller (1976) and Creaghead, Newman, and Secord (1989) suggest that the following events are developed: (1) the ability to control the vocal mechanism by turning it on and off at will; (2) control of variations and extremes of pitch; (3) control of volume of vocalization; (4) control of resonance; (5) control of timing of speech production and vocal tract resonance and constriction, in order to differentiate vowels and consonants, differentiate voice and voiceless cognates, and produce syllables rapidly and accurately.

Underlying the developmental progression from communicative intent to the use of words is the maturation of the mechanism that produces sounds.

■ The Neonate

No other human organ system needs to work as immediately and effectively as the larynx. Because of its integrated physiologic relationship to the entire airway, the larynx must immediately serve as both an air conduit and protector of the lower airway (Fried 1988; Kamen 1989).

At birth, the larynx is located at the level of the third cervical vertebra. During swallowing, the larynx may rise as high as the first or second cervical vertebral body. The infant's larynx differs from the adult's in shape and in proximity of its extralaryngeal structures. The high position of the larynx is retained for the first six months of life and permits highly efficient airflow due to decreased airway resistance. Continuous with the oral-pharyngeal cavity, the mucosa of the laryngeal cavity is richly supplied with sensory receptors that are mature at the cellular level (Bosma 1985). The airway configuration of the adult is relatively straight and inferior to the base of the tongue, and the epiglottis is in similar vertical alignment to the trachea. In contrast, the infant's airway configuration is more curved from the oral cavity through the larynx into the trachea (Eavey 1988). Furthermore, the infant airway is comprised of more pliable connective tissue. As a result, normal pressures generated during respiration can cause deformity of the airway. (Refer to diagrams of the newborn infant's oral and pharyngeal mechanisms in Chapter 2.)

The thyroid cartilage in the neonate is semicircular, with the two laminae meeting at a 130-degree angle. It is located in an inferior and posterior position relative to the hyoid bone (Eckenroth 1951; Cote and Todres 1985). Arytenoid cartilages in the neonate have limited mobility due to a thick mucosal covering and to their large size in comparison to the laryngeal cavity. As the child matures, the arytenoid cartilages undergo little change in gross dimensions, but adapt in form (Klock and Beckwith 1985; Eavey 1988). The hyoid bone of the neonate overlaps the thyroid.

Fried, Kelly, and Strome (1982) and Tucker (1980) reported that the cricoid cartilage is the most prominent vocal tract cartilage during the first three months of life. This cartilage is ovoid in shape, and its inferior-posterior orientation gives the subglottic airway its funnel-like appearance (Klock and Beckwith 1985). Consequently, the diameter of the subglottic airway is less than that of the airway above the glottis. The length of the vocal folds and ventricular folds is large in comparison to the internal dimensions of the thyroid and cricoid cartilages (Bosma 1975; Ardran and Kemp 1970). In the neonate, the length of the vocal folds is six to eight millimeters and the subglottic anteroposterior diameter, considered the critical dimension of the infant larynx, is approximately five to seven millimeters (Tucker 1980).

Motor and sensory information obtained during postural and movement control provide the basis for normal speech motor control. According to Kent (1976), Bosma (1975), and Netsell (1982), speech motor control is evidenced in the increased spatial and temporal coordination of the articulatory structures within the oral-pharyngeal and laryngeal cavities. Neural and musculoskeletal development of these structures is essential to the achievement of vocal tract control for generation of the systematic and repeatable acoustic variations perceived as speech.

From birth to three months of age, major neural connections are being formed and completed in the pre- and post-thalamic and optic tracts. Upper motor neuron myelination of the corticospinal and corticobulbar tracts and post-thalamic auditory and somatosensory pathways also occurs during this period. According to Milner (1976) and Netsell (1980), upper motor and sensory areas are fairly well developed. This suggests that some newborn movement patterns are initiated at the cortical level. Association areas are nonfunctional during this time. Primitive reflexes are not inhibited and remain so until the third month when cortical inhibition is activated (Capute 1978).

Although capable of sound production, the infant's vocal tract is better suited for respiration during the first three months of life. Speech involves supralaryngeal vocal tract filtering of sounds generated by air turbulence and/or vocal fold vibration (Chiba and Kajiyama 1941; Fant 1960; Lieberman 1977). During speech production, the continually changing shape of the supralaryngeal vocal tract (for example, oral and pharyngeal cavities) alters its resonant properties, and, therefore, the nature of the filter.

Anatomically, the infant vocal tract lacks clearly defined oral and pharyngeal cavities due to approximation of the soft palate and epiglottis, filling of the oral cavity by the tongue, and the high position of the larynx and hyoid bone (Lieberman 1977; Bosma 1975; DuBrul 1977; Laitman and Crelin 1976). Consequently, the resonant properties differ from those of an anatomically mature vocal tract.

The relationship of the hard palate to the basicranium is a significant landmark of the infant vocal tract. The hard palate and velum are located in a more superior position than is seen in the adult. At birth, positioning of the velum and orientation of its extrinsic musculature limit the capacity of the velum to function effectively in regulating oral versus nasal airflow (Bosma and Fletcher 1961; Bosma 1975). In addition, there appears to be no well defined pharyngeal portion in the direct airway when the velum occludes the nasal cavity (Lieberman 1977).

As discussed earlier, the oral space of the newborn infant is small, partly due to the size of the mandible. The lower jaw remains slightly retracted until four to six months of age when a downward growth of the mandible creates a larger intraoral space. The tongue is also limited in its ability to function as an articulator since, at rest, the tongue of the newborn infant completely fills the oral cavity. Its short anterior-posterior dimension and wide lateral dimension creates a "clumsy articulator." In addition, the size of the tongue relative to the volume of the oral cavity limits the resonating capacity of the cavity (Kamen 1989).

From the neonatal period through the third month of life, the anatomical structures and the alignment of the oral-pharyngeal and laryngeal cavities constitute a relatively constrained resonant system. Therefore, sounds of the neonate are nasally resonated. The small oral cavity, filled with the tongue, and the high position of the larynx and hyoid bone leave the nasal cavity as the only effective resonator.

The neonate is capable of expressive communication well before formal verbal language is developed. McLean and Snyder-McLean (1978) suggested that the infant communicates pre-linguistically for the following reasons: relief of discomfort; reestablishment of proximity; attainment of desired ends; and initiation, maintenance, and termination of an interaction. Although neonates are limited in the behaviors they can use for communication, the maturity of the facial neuromuscular system allows them to use facial expression to communicate displeasure, fear, joy, and anger (Owens 1988). The infant responds differentially to the caretaker's face and voice by as early as two weeks of age, and by three weeks, the social smile (not dependent upon the infant's internal physical state) is observed. Vocal interaction with the environment is limited to reflexive rather than volitional cognitive communicative acts. However, crying, whimpering, sneezing, grunting, sucking, yawning, sighing, gooing, and cooing are pre-linguistic in nature. The beginnings of intention of communication observed in neonates through body tension, posturing, eye gaze, and head movement are all precursors to intentional communication. According to Kaye (1979), by the time infants have developed the representational and phonemic systems to begin learning language, they are already able to make their intentions understood (most of the time), can elicit repetitions and variations, and are able to understand and interpret others' responses.

Motor control develops in reference to this neuroanatomic scheme. The most prevalent motor act of the newborn infant is crying. The neonatal cry is a life supporting action. Its cause may be hunger or pain/discomfort and is a signal for attention. Wilder and Baken (1974), Langlois and Baken (1976), and Wilder and Baken (1978), report that the infant cry follows its own developmental course related to anatomic modifications of respiratory, laryngeal, and oral structures. Speech-like sounds are heard within the cry. Front vowels ($\varepsilon/\text{æ}/e/i/$) are most common and back vowels are almost entirely absent. In addition, distress cries tend to be more consonant-like or fricated whereas non-distress cries use respiratory-laryngeal controls similar to those associated with primarily vocalic, short duration expiratory vocalizations. These vocalizations are position dependent and are elicited without interruption by rib cage or abdominal movements (Baken 1979; Hixon 1973).

■ One to Two Months

Although the sounds of a child's native language are acquired within the first four years of life, well before the onset of the first word, the child begins to recognize that sound conveys information and that certain sounds evoke varied responses within the environment. From birth to three months communicative intent is marked by shared rhythms between parent and child (Kaye 1982). The "dialogue" is developed from the regularity of sucking-attention-arousal cycles. By two months of age, the beginnings of "shared intentions" are observed. The infant begins to use a behavior that once attracted attention (for example, coughing) as an initiator of an exchange.

Two months marks the beginning of subjectivity, whereby the infant demonstrates a distinctive behavior towards people that is different from that towards objects (Owens 1988). The sharing begins unilaterally, where the parent guesses at the intentions of the infant's behaviors. Often the parent attributes more elaborate meanings to the intent, such as relating cries to the physiological states of hunger or pain, or restless fatigue movements are interpreted as though the signs were the intent to do something about the state. That is, the parent labels the context and thereby integrates the child into an already existing social environment. Relative to the cognitive and perceptual bases of language development, it is contextual representations and associations that give words and symbols meaning.

■ Three to Five Months

During the first three months of life, infants learn that their signals yield a response. This marks the beginning of infants' impressions of their control of the environment, dependent on the degree of parental response. By four months of age, the infant develops rituals and game-playing behaviors (Trevarthen and Hubley 1978). Predictable patterns of speech and behavior can be observed during feeding, changing, and bedtime. Games such as "peek-a-boo," "I'm gonna get you," "piggy," or "pat-a-cake" provide the opportunity for turn taking, the learning of rules, and pauses that permit reactions or words to eventually be interjected. This partnership of exchanges fosters dialogue. Five months marks an increase in the child's ability to imitate movements and vocalizations. These vocalizations are often demonstrative of emotion (happy, sad, angry, eager), and are voiced to people, toys, and mirror images.

Myelination of the pyramidal tract, corticobulbar and corticospinal tracts, and post-thalamic auditory and somatosensory pathways occurs between three and twelve months of age. Major development is observed in the middle cerebellar peduncle, considered to be a key cerebellar area in speech motor control (Yakolev and Lecours 1967).

Vegetative sounds (coughing, belching, sneezing) as well as crying and cooing vocalizations during the first three months are limited by anatomic constraints and overall instability of the vocal tract. Although both voiced and voiceless sounds are produced, Stark, Rose, and McLagen (1975) reported that approximately 30 percent of vegetative sounds are voiceless and are produced on either inspiration or expiration. However, cooing and crying sounds are produced on expiration and are voiced.

Due to apposition of the laryngeal and nasopharyngeal cavities, most consonantal sounds are produced by alternating velar to uvular constriction. The sounds /g/, /n/, and /ŋ/ are heard primarily in supine and represent the beginning of systematic alternations of vocal tract opening and closing gestures (Stark 1979; Oller 1978; Morris 1978, 1982). Bilabial sound play is observed in prone, and the emergence of alveolar sounds is evident in a supported sitting position.

Because of the anatomic relationship between the tongue and the jaw, infants most frequently produce high front or central vowels. Low back vowels are produced approximately 25 percent of the time. The poorly defined pharyngeal region in the first three to four months of life also restricts the magnitude of tongue displacements in all directions.

In considering vowel production, Lieberman (1977) reported that the supralaryngeal vocal tract of the adult approximates a "two-tubed" resonating system. To produce the vowels /i/, /ɑ/, /u/, distinct perceptual boundaries of vocal tract configurations must be approximated at the oral-pharyngeal junction. Adults are able to produce these configurations by maintaining a midpoint of constriction and independently manipulating the volume of the oral-pharyngeal cavities. In contrast, the anatomy of the infant limits the range of possible vowel types. In addition, this "single-tubed" resonating system restricts the range of configurations for vowel production. As a result, the infant is able to achieve only cross-sectional area cavity changes by distortions of the tongue body in the oral cavity (Lieberman 1977).

By the fourth month, increases in intraoral space and elongation of the pharyngeal cavity give rise to increases in the variety of vocalic sounds. Furthermore, greater anterior-posterior space and increased separation of the oral and nasal cavities is created by downward and forward growth of the mandible, downward shift of the larynx and hyoid, and separation of the epiglottis and soft palate.

Morse (1972) suggested that as the spatial organization of the vocal tract changes during the fourth month, the infant continually explores, maps, and updates sensory information through touch, pressure, and movement within the oral-pharyngeal cavity. Bosma (1975) indicated that coincident with pharyngeal cavity surface area enlargement and reduction of sensory receptors in the oral-pharyngeal mucosa, there is heightened sensory reception to touch, pressure, and movement of the lip margins and tongue tip.

The lips, tongue, and jaw play a more active role as infants develop independent control of their movements. Emergence of tongue blade elevation and increased range of motion produces a variety of sounds that are independent of tongue body position. Approximation of the tongue to the soft palate, tongue to the alveolar ridge, and tongue to lips, as well as bilabial contact, produces cavity sources of frication on expiration (Stark 1979). Although the majority of consonants produced at this time are velar sounds, bilabials and "raspberry" lip frication and smacking sounds are emerging. This represents the beginning of front-to-back contrast of the articulators within a newly opened front of the vocal tract (Oller 1978; Stark 1979; Morris 1978, 1982; Alexander 1982).

Articulatory-phonetic output of the developing child is, therefore, directly related to anatomic and physiologic changes. Structural changes of the oral-pharyngeal cavity directly influence its filtering capacity as well as facilitate an increased variety of discrete movements of the articulators. In addition, the laryngeal cavity structures support multiple physiologic roles that change with development. The early double-tubed structural configuration fosters optimal performance of respiration and alimentation. By three months of age, respiration and alimentation functions are performed by a single-tubed structural system. Beginning at six months, the onset of greater excursions of the laryngeal structures and changes in the length and mass of the vocal folds permit changes in the acoustic output, which continue through puberty.

Breathing patterns change in the four- to six-month-old infant because of the loss of apposition of the soft palate and epiglottis. In addition, the junction of the nasal pathway and lower respiratory structures begins to change in contour to the right angle observed in adults. The double-tubed system present in the first three months changes to a single-tubed respiratory/alimentary system. Oral and oral-nasal breathing are present, and swallowing now involves active closure of the vocal folds and active descent of the epiglottis to protect the airway. The creation of a single-tubed system will have major effects on the acoustic properties of the infant's phonatory output.

■ Six to Twelve Months

During the second half of the first year of life, infants begin to take more control of their interactions with the environment. They develop the ability to communicate their intentions with greater efficiency and effect. By eight to nine months of age, the baby imitates simple motor acts such as waving bye-bye on request. Also at this time, babies develop intentionality (Owens 1988). They no longer have to focus on only an object or a person. They can now use gesture as a functional signalling system, such as getting an adult's attention and gesturing what is desired. By 12 months of age, words accompany or replace gesture as a means of meaningful speech and communication.

The 3- to 12-month period marks a transition in motor control from neonate to more adult-like patterns characterized by the emergence of efferent, afferent, auditory, movement, and somatosensory routines that subserve adult speech motor control (Netsell 1980). For example, as mentioned earlier, the infant's acquisition of antigravity control effects mandibular growth in a downward and forward direction as well as effecting downward movement of the larynx (Moyers 1971; Kent 1979, 1982). Further, the mandible-hyoid-laryngeal suspensions develop as the upper airway assumes adult dimensions. Finally, from the immature pump-like suck-swallow and suckle patterns emerges the more mature swallow exhibiting tongue retraction and independent lip and jaw mobility. (Refer to the diagram of the adult oral and pharyngeal mechanisms in Chapter 7.)

By the time the infant reaches the 12- to 24-month period, considerable growth occurs in the middle and anterior sections of the neocortex (Milner 1976). Myelination of the corpus striatum begins in the ninth month. This area is responsible for postural and movement control. Desmedt (1978) suggests that, taken as a composite, these neural-cortical connections form the network of circuits (loops) underlying fine motor control.

As primitive reflex patterns become inhibited cortically, neural organization is observed in EEG activity (Milner 1976; Woodruff 1978). Full myelination of post-thalamic somesthetic pathways is not complete until 18 months of age. Myelination of these pathways puts the cerebellar-cortical motor pathways into action so that the emerging movement patterns for speech can be practiced using a full range of the fast- acting cortical, cerebellar, somatosensory, and corticothalamic loops (Desmedt 1978). Gazzanga (1970) noted that good interhemispheric function is not apparent until two to three years of age. Post-thalamic auditory pathways are continuing to undergo myelination. Cortical layers are developing vertically with respect to the neural axis. Horizontal connections between association areas are just beginning to undergo myelination. These connections, along with connections of the commissures, grow rapidly and are completely myelinated at the end of the seventh year (Yakolev and Lecours 1967).

As a result of separation of the epiglottis from the larynx and soft palate, the epiglottis can no longer passively protect the airway during feeding. Food now passes over the epiglottis instead of around its lateral borders. The protective role of the larynx during deglutition is established at this time. That is, the larynx and the hyoid must actively move the now descended structures closer to the epiglottis. The epiglottis, in turn, moves downward and backward to protect the airway (Logan and Bosma 1967; Logemann 1985). Thus, the protective function of the larynx during swallowing begins at this time and is mediated by: (1) descent of the epiglottis, (2) medial approximation of the ventricular and true vocal folds, and (3) elevation of the hyoid and larynx.

Eruption of the first teeth changes the vertical dimension of the oral cavity. This change fosters greater range of tongue movement, including the beginning of independent tongue tip elevation during the swallow. Eruption of the first molars also brings about anatomical change. That is, there is an increase in posterior and transverse dimensions of the oral cavity. By the end of the first year of life, functional anatomic changes within the oral-pharyngeal and laryngeal cavities are complete. Refinement will continue through puberty.

By six months of age, the infant is producing /m/, /p/, /b/, /n/, and /w/. As greater control of the palatal levator develops, the infant demonstrates velopharyngeal differentiation of consonant sounds sharing the same place of articulation (for example, bilabial /b/ versus bilabial nasal /m/). Furthermore, greater variety in vowel production and the emergence of voiced alveolar sounds are evident. Babbling, observed for the first time at this six-month stage, is highly variable in rate and rhythm. In addition, first stages of syllabification are noted in the production of prolonged glides and diphthongs (Zlatin and Koenigsknecht 1975; Stark 1979).

By seven to nine months of age, anatomic maturation of the orbicularis oris muscle (the last of the facial muscles to mature) and eruption of the lateral incisors effect increased control and differentiation of lip movements and provide a new set of sensory receptors. Additional evidence of motor control is the appearance of rhythm as a basis of speed and precision of speech production during reduplicated babbling (Morris 1982). Reduplicated babbling requires respiratory support adequate to produce prolonged bursts of phonation and sufficient motor control to produce rhythmical opening and closing of the oral cavity (Stark 1979; Morris 1978, 1982). The consonant and vowel combinations produced in reduplicated babbling contain the same consonant in every syllable.

During the seven- to nine-month period, the primary place of articulation shifts from velar to lingual-alveolar, followed by labial. Frequency of velar placement of articulation decreases to approximately 15 percent of total output (Oller 1978; Stark

1979; Morris 1978). The most prevalent consonant types produced are stops, nasals, and /j/ glides. Although production of fricatives and affricates may emerge by eight months of age, they are produced in isolation (not in combination with a vowel). By nine months, precise voluntary release of consonant constriction is observed in stop consonant-vowel combinations and in the adult-like durations of the syllable and consonant-vowel transitions (Stark 1979). Furthermore, all vowels and diphthongs produced are fully resonant.

Beginning at the ninth to tenth month of development, variegated babbling replaces reduplicated babbling. The infant is able to produce long chains of different consonant-vowel combinations. Consonants that were present in reduplicated babbling are also present in this non-reduplicated babbling phase. This period of development is thought to designate the beginning of imitation. Making an association of auditory and motor events, the child now spontaneously and imitatively vocalizes familiar sound patterns heard in the environment (Oller 1976; Stark 1979). Fricative (/s/, /z/, / ʃ/, /tʃ /, /f/ and /v/) and vowel combinations are now added to the sound repertoire, but are inconsistent in frequency of occurrence. This sound combination is more difficult than the stop-consonant plus vowel combination as it requires a higher level of motor control to sustain the narrow constriction of the oral cavity necessary for generating turbulent airflow (Stark 1979). Bilabials, labio-dentals, and alveolars comprise approximately 80 percent of the consonants produced. Velars make up the remaining 20 percent.

Changes in vowel production are also observed during this stage of development. Production of high front as well as mid and high back rounded and unrounded vowels emerges as a result of increased volume of the oral cavity.

During the transition from babbling to first words from 12 months through 18 months of age, stress and intonation patterns (jargon) are evident. Eruption of first molars and incisors increase the vertical dimension of the oral cavity, giving rise to more vertical space for tongue movement. In addition, independent control of jaw and tongue movements is now observed consistently. Alveolar consonants make up almost 70 percent of the consonant repertoire, while labial and velar consonants occur approximately 15 percent of the time. High, mid, and low vowels are used in equal proportion, but back vowels are still produced infrequently. Front and central vowels are produced with greatest frequency.

For the first year of life, the anatomy of the oral-pharyngeal and laryngeal cavities support survival of the neurologically and motorically immature infant by providing structural stability and passive regulation of functions that will later require greater motor coordination. Further, the slowly evolving anatomic changes interact with neurologic development to give rise to functional changes. That is, functional maturation can be attributed to anatomical changes in conjunction with neurological maturation for motor control. Thus, it appears that normal functional experiences and refinement of function through these experiences can occur only in the context of a normal progression of anatomic and neurologic development.

Kent (1979) designated the 24-month period as the time when development of spatial coordination is completed. At this time, vocal tract shaping and articulatory coordination are adequate to produce sequences of different speech sounds. During this period, the primary neurological maturation necessary for coordination and motor control of movement patterns, anatomic growth necessary for cavity shaping, and practice influences on precision of articulatory placement are integrated to produce predictable (stable) and recognizable speech acoustic output.

The child now combines two or more words using the entire range of vowels and diphthongs and consonants. However, speech movements are slower and consonant-vowel segment durations are more variable than in adults. Beyond 24 months, development of speech production emphasizes temporal aspects of motor control. This will continue until puberty.

By the third year of life, the oral-pharyngeal anatomy of the vocal tract resembles that of the adult in the following manner: (1) presence of a short, broad cavity, (2) right angle bend of the oral-pharyngeal channel, (3) a long pharyngeal cavity, (4) posterior aspect of the tongue dorsum, (5) deeply recessed larynx, and (6) separation of the epiglottis and soft palate. Developmental anatomic changes fostered changes in function and provided the framework upon which maturation of motor control, resulting in variations in output, and practice in articulator movement (through vegetative functions, feeding, and vocal play) are imposed to result in the development of speech.

■ Summary

Articulatory-phonetic output of the developing child is directly related to anatomic and physiologic changes. Structural changes of the oral-pharyngeal cavity directly influence its filtering capacity as well as facilitate increased variety of discrete movements of the articulators. In addition, the laryngeal cavity structures support multiple physiologic roles that change with development. The early double-tubed structural configuration fosters optimal performance of respiration and alimentation. By three months of age, respiration and alimentation functions are performed by a single-tubed structural system. Beginning at six months, the onset of greater excursions of the laryngeal structures and changes in length and mass of the vocal folds permit changes in the acoustic output, which continue through puberty.

The emergence of words coincides with the completion of myelination of a majority of sensorimotor pathways and stabilization of musculoskeletal growth. Oral, pharyngeal, and laryngeal structures at this time move in synchrony but at a slower rate than in the adult. Longer durations are observed in the uttered word or word approximations made up of simple consonant-vowel syllabic structures.

Speech refinement occurs from 2 to 14 years of age. Myelination of the cerebellar peduncle, post-thalamic acoustic pathways, and cerebral commissures is complete by the end of the second year. Associated areas continue to undergo myelination through the third decade of life. Modification of inter-articulator timing and vocal tract shape begins at approximately three years of age. As spatial and temporal coordination increase, an increase in overall speech motor control is evident in the ability to vary the spatial relations of the oral, pharyngeal, and laryngeal cavities. As a result, variations of manner and place of articulation are facilitated (Kent 1976).

Development of a motor skill is not an isolated process. Every aspect of motor control proceeds from gross patterns to highly refined motor coordination patterns. In reference to the speech mechanism, the infant is initially restricted in movement by anatomy and immature neural development. The oral structures at birth move in gross patterns and the more adult-like function of the laryngeal structures does not emerge for almost six months. As development progresses, gross oral movement patterns give rise to independent movements of the anatomical structures. Furthermore, this independence appears in conjunction with increased neuromotor development and produces the more refined oral motor control needed for the fine gradients of pressure, contact, and posturing required for speech.

■ References

Alexander, R. 1982. Early feeding, sound production, and pre-linguistic/cognitive development and their relationship to gross motor and fine motor development. Unpublished working document, Milwaukee, Wisconsin.

Ardran, G., and F. Kemp. 1970. Some important factors in the assessment of oral-pharyngeal function. *Developmental Medicine and Child Neurology* 12:158-66.

Baken, R. J. 1979. Acoustics and perception of infant cry. In *Infant cry*, edited by C. Murray. New York: Academic Press.

Bosma, J. 1975. Anatomic and physiologic development of the speech apparatus. In *Human communications and its disorders*, Vol. 3, edited by D. Tower, 469-81. New York: Raven Press.

_____. 1985. Postnatal ontogeny of performances of the pharynx, larynx, and mouth. *American Review of Respiratory Disorders* 131 (Suppl): 510-15.

Bosma, J., and S. Fletcher. 1961. Comparison of pharyngeal action in infant cry and mature phonation. *Logos* 4:100-17.

Capute, J. 1978. Primitive reflex profile. In *Monographs in developmental pediatrics*, Vol. 1. Baltimore: University Park Press.

Chiba, T. S., and M. Kajiyama. 1941. *The vowel: Its nature and structure.* Tokyo: Kaiseikan, Tokyo.

Cote, C., and I. D. Todres. 1985. The pediatric airway. In *A practice of anesthesiology for infants and children*, edited by J. F. Ryan, 35-57. Orlando, FL: Grune & Stratton.

Creaghead, N., P. Newman, and W. Secord. 1989. *Assessment and remediation of articulatory and phonological disorders* (2nd edition). Columbus, OH: Merrill Publishing.

Desmedt, J. 1978. In *Cerebral motor control in man: Long loop mechanism*, edited by S. Karger. New York: Academic Press.

DuBrul, E. 1977. Biomechanics of speech sounds. *Annals of New York Academy of Sciences* 280:631-42.

Eavey, R. D. 1988. The pediatric larynx. In *The larynx: A multidisciplinary approach*, edited by M. P. Fried, 31-40. Boston: Little Brown & Co.

Eckenroth, J. E. 1951. Some anatomic considerations of the infant larynx influencing endotracheal anesthesia. *Anesthesiology* 12:401.

Fant, G. 1960. *Acoustic theory of speech production*. The Hague: Mouton.

Fried, M. P. 1988. *The larynx: A multidisciplinary approach*. New York: Ravens Press.

Fried, M. P., J. H. Kelly, and M. Strome. 1982. Comparison of the adult and infant larynx. *Journal of Family Practice* 15:557.

Gazzanga, M. 1970. *The bisected brain*. New York: Appleton.

Hixon, T. 1973. Respiratory function in speech. In *Normal aspects of speech, hearing, and language*, edited by F. Minifie, T. Hixon, and S. Williams, 73-126. Englewood Cliffs, NJ: Prentice Hall, Inc.

Kamen, R. Saletsky. 1989. Effects of long-term tracheotomy on selected spectral and temporal indices of speech production development. Ph.D. diss. University of Texas at Dallas. In *Dissertation abstracts international* 50(09, Sec B: 900-3990):3949.

Kaye, K. 1979. Thickening thin data: The maternal role in developing communication and language. In *Before speech*, edited by M. Bullowa. New York: Cambridge University Press.

_____. 1982. *Social interaction of language and learning*. New York: Academic Press.

Kent, R. D. 1976. Tutorial-anatomic and neuromuscular maturation of the speech mechanism: Evidence from acoustic studies. *Journal of Speech and Hearing Research* 19:421-47.

———. 1979. Articulatory-acoustic perspectives on speech development. Johnson and Johnson conference on language behavior in infancy and early childhood. Santa Barbara, CA.

———. 1982. Sensorimotor aspects of speech development. In *Development of Perception*, Vol. 1, edited by R. N. Aslin, J. R. Alberts, and M. R. Peterson. New York: Academic Press.

Klock, E., and J. Beckwith. 1985. Dimensions of the human larynx during infancy and childhood. In *Anatomy of the newborn head*, edited by J. Bosma, 368-71. Baltimore: Johns Hopkins Press.

Laitman, J. T., and E. S. Crelin. 1976. Postnatal development of the basicranium and vocal tract region in man. In *Symposium on development of the basicranium*, edited by J. D. Bosma. Bethesda, MD: National Institutes of Health (DHEW Pub. NIH-76-989).

Langlois, A., and R. Baken. 1976. Development of respiratory factors in infant cry. *Developmental Medicine and Child Neurology* 18:732-37.

Lieberman, P. 1977. *Speech physiology and acoustic phonetics*. New York: Macmillan Publishing.

Logan, W. J., and J. Bosma. 1967. Oral and pharyngeal dysphagia in infancy. *Pediatric Clinics of North America* 14:47-61.

Logemann, J. 1985. *Swallowing and swallowing disorders*. Baltimore: College Hill Press.

McLean, J., and L. Snyder-McLean. 1978. *A transactional approach to early language training*. Columbus, OH: Merrill Publishing.

Milner, E. 1976. CNS maturation and language acquisition. In *Studies in neurolinguistics*, Vol. 1, edited by H. Whitaker and H. A. Whitaker. New York: Academic Press.

Morris, S. E. 1978. Treatment of children with oral-motor dysfunction. In *Oral-motor function and dysfunction in children*, edited by J. M. Wilson, 163-85. Chapel Hill, NC: University of North Carolina.

———. 1982. *The normal acquisition of oral feeding skills: Implications for assessment and treatment*. Santa Barbara, CA: Therapeutic Media.

Morse, P. 1972. The discrimination of speech and non-speech stimuli in early infancy. *Journal of Experimental Child Psychology* 14:447-92.

Moyers, R. E. 1971. Postnatal development of the orofacial musculature. *ASHA Reports* 6:38-47.

Netsell, R. 1980. The acquisition of speech motor control: A perspective with directions for research. Paper presented at convention. American Speech-Language-Hearing Association, Detroit, MI.

_____. 1982. Speech motor control and selected neurological disorders. In *Speech motor control*, Vol. 36, edited by S. Grillner, B. Lindblom, and J. Persson. New York: Pergamon Press.

Oller, D. K. 1976. Analysis of infant vocalizations. Miniseminar presented at convention. American Speech-Language-Hearing Association, Houston.

_____. 1978. Infant vocalization and the development of speech. *Allied Health and Behavior Science* 1:523-49.

Owens, R. E. 1988. *Language development* (2nd edition). Columbus, OH: Merrill Publishing.

Stark, R. E. 1979. Pre-speech segmental feature development. In *Language acquisition*, edited by Fletcher and Garman. Cambridge, MA: Cambridge University Press.

Stark, R. E., S. N. Rose, and M. McLagen. 1975. Features of infant sounds: The first eight weeks of life. *Journal of Child Language* 2(2):205-22.

Trevarthen, C., and P. Hubley. 1978. Secondary intersubjectivity: Confidence, confiding, and acts of meaning in the first year of life. In *Action, gesture and symbol: The emergence of language*, edited by A. Lock. New York: Academic Press.

Tucker, H. 1980. Laryngeal development and congenital lesions. *Annals of Otolaryngology, Rhinology, and Laryngology* 74(Suppl.):142-45.

Wilder, C. N., and R. J. Baken. 1974. Respiratory patterns in infant cry. *Human Communication*. Winter: 18-34.

_____. 1978. Some developmental aspects of infancy. *Journal of Genetic Psychology* 132:225-30.

Woodruff, R. 1978. Brain electrical activities and behavior: Relationships over the lifespan. In *Lifespan development and behavior*, edited by P. Bates. New York: Academic Press.

Yakolev, P., and A. Lecours. 1967. The myelogenetic cycles of regional maturation of the brain. In *Regional development of the brain in early life*, edited by R. Minkowski. Oxford, England: Blackwell Scientific Publications.

Zlatin, M. A., and R. A. Koenigsknecht. 1975. Development of voicing contrast: A comparison of voice onset time in stop perception and production. *Journal of Speech and Hearing Research* 19:93-111.

Glossary

Abdominal muscles. Muscles of the abdominal wall, including the external and internal obliques, the transversus abdominus, the rectus abdominus, and the quadratus lumborum, with primary roles in active antigravity trunk flexion and stabilizing the lower rib cage during respiration.

Abdominal-thoracic breathing. A respiratory pattern characterized by expansion of the thoracic and upper abdominal areas on inhalation; the rib cage elevates as it expands laterally and in the anterior-posterior dimension, while the diaphragm contracts and lowers, creating expansion vertically.

Abduction. A movement of a limb part away from the center of the body.

Acromioclavicular joint. Relating to both the acromial process of the scapula and its articulation with the clavicle.

Adduction. A movement of a limb part toward the center of the body.

Asymmetrical tonic neck reflex. Not really a reflex, but a reaction or postural response in which rotation of the head results in a "fencing" pattern of the upper extremities with flexion of the elbow on the skull side and extension on the face side.

Automatic phasic bite-release pattern. A response to tactile input presented to the biting surfaces of the gums or teeth; composed of a small, rhythmical series of up/down jaw movements; occurs until approximately 5 months of age.

Automatic stepping. A newborn reaction elicited by placing the infant upright on the feet, which results in a walking pattern.

Belly breathing. A respiratory pattern in which the diaphragm contracts and pushes against the abdominal wall resulting in belly expansion and flaring of the lower ribs as air is taken in on inhalation; diaphragmatic or abdominal breathing.

Bilateral reach. The simultaneous use of both upper extremities in reach.

Bimanual dexterity. The ability to involve each hand in a different motor task within the same function, such as cutting meat.

Binocular fixation. The ability to use both eyes simultaneously to focus on a target and fuse the two images into a single perception.

Buccal fat pads. See Sucking pads.

Buccinator muscle. The major paired facial muscle of the cheeks that courses forward from the pterygomandibular raphe, superior pharyngeal constrictor, and alveolar processes of the mandible and maxilla to the mucous membrane of the cheeks and the orbicularis oris and skin of the lips; pulls the corners of the lips laterally and posteriorly for lip spreading; makes cheeks taut when mouth opens and closes as in sucking, chewing, and swallowing.

Caudal. Directed toward the lower body or feet.

Cephalic. Directed toward the head.

Chewing. The process used to break up solid foods in preparation for swallowing.

Constrictor muscles. Muscles of the lateral and posterior walls of the pharynx; the superior, middle, and inferior pharyngeal constrictors make the walls of the pharynx mobile; on contraction, they constrict the pharyngeal cavity, creating peristaltic movement to propel food to the esophagus.

Controlled, sustained bite. The easy, graded closure of the teeth through a solid food with an easy, graded release for chewing.

Deciduous teeth. The 20 temporary or primary teeth that develop from about 6 months through 24-30 months of age.

Deltoids. A group of muscles that act on the humerus. The anterior portions flex, horizontally adduct, and internally rotate the humerus. The middle portion abducts the humerus to 90 degrees. The posterior portion extends, horizontally abducts, and externally rotates the humerus.

Diaphragm. The musculotendinous sheet that separates the thoracic and abdominal cavities; its muscle fibers arise from the inner surfaces of the sternum and lower ribs and from the bodies of the upper lumbar vertebrae to insert on its central tendon; during inhalation, the central tendon is pulled down and forward as the lower ribs are pulled up and outward, and the sternum is raised, vertically increasing the thoracic cavity and pushing the abdominal wall outward.

Dorsiflexion. A movement of the foot towards the anterior aspect of the lower leg.

Dynamic scapular stability. The ability of muscles acting on the scapula to keep it stable on the thorax during its movement on the thorax.

Epiglottis. The thin fibrocartilaginous structure covered by a thick submucosa at the uppermost aspect of the larynx.

Equilibrium reactions. Complex feedback-type postural reactions elicited by an unexpected movement of the body's center of mass that perturbs balance.

Erector spinae. A group of deep muscles of the back that, when contracting bilaterally, extend the spine or maintain it in an erect position; when contracting unilaterally, some muscles can laterally bend those segments of the spine they are attached to and others may rotate the vertebrae.

Esophagus. The musculomembranous tube extending from the pharynx to the stomach.

Eversion. A lateral movement of the plantar surface of the foot directing it away from midline.

Exhalation. The part of the respiratory cycle when air is forced out of the lungs; expiration.

Extension. A straightening or backward movement of the spine or limbs.

External rotation. An outward turning of a limb away from the body.

Extrinsic tongue muscles. Four muscles that provide a framework for stability and move the tongue; the fibers of the genioglossus, styloglossus, palatoglossus, and hyoglossus originate from the mandible, styloid process of the temporal bone, soft palate, and hyoid bone, respectively, and insert into the tongue.

Eye convergence. Directing the visual axis of two eyes to a near point.

Faucial arches. Anterior and posterior faucial pillars formed by the palatoglossus and palatopharyngeus muscles at the posterior border of the oral cavity; they play a role in lowering the soft palate.

Feeding. A process that refers to the child's environment, parent-child interactions, the medical, developmental, neuromotor, sensory-motor, and cognitive integrity of the child, feeding techniques, feeding utensils, positioning needs, swallowing, the interaction of swallowing with respiratory and gastrointestinal factors, and the child's nutritional requirements.

Femoral angle. The angle formed by the neck and shaft of the femur.

Flexion. A bending or forward movement of the spine or limbs.

Gag response. A response to tactile input presented to the back of the tongue or oropharyngeal area composed of jaw extension, forward/downward tongue movement, and pharyngeal constriction.

Glenohumeral joint. Relating to the glenoid cavity and the humeral head.

Glenoid fossa. The cavity of the scapula forming the shoulder joint and articulating with the humeral head.

Grasp reflex. A flexion response that occurs when an object is placed in the hand.

Grip strength. The ability to grasp an object and maintain it against resistance.

Hamstrings. A muscle group of the posterior thigh that can flex the knee and extend the hip.

Hard palate. The bony palate or roof of the mouth formed by the palatine processes of the maxilla and the palatine bones.

Horizontal adduction. Movement of the arm toward or beyond midline at approximately a 90-degree plane.

Humeral abduction. Movement of the upper arm away from the lateral aspect of the trunk.

Humeral adduction. Movement of the upper arm toward the lateral aspect of the trunk.

Humeral extension. Movement of the upper arm behind the trunk.

Humeral external rotation. A turning outward or laterally of the upper arm.

Humeral flexion. Movement of the upper arm away from the anterior aspect of the trunk.

Humeral internal rotation. A turning inward or medially of the upper arm.

Hyoid bone. The small bone suspended within the pharynx by the suprahyoid and infrahyoid muscles without any other bony attachments; through its musculature attachments it influences tongue, jaw, and laryngeal function.

Iliopsoas. A muscle group consisting of the psoas and the iliacus; the combined action is flexion/abduction/external rotation of the hip. The upper portion of the psoas can also extend the thoraco-lumbar area of the spine.

Infrahyoid muscles. The four, paired "strap" muscles, including the sternothyroid and thyrohyoid (connect the sternum and first rib to the thyroid and connect the thyroid to the hyoid), the omohyoid (courses from the scapula to the hyoid), and the sternohyoid (connects the sternum and clavicle to the hyoid); these muscles assist in depressing the hyoid and work with the suprahyoids to fix the hyoid in position and to flex the head.

Inhalation. The part of the respiratory cycle when air is brought into the lungs.

Intercostal muscles. The external intercostals course diagonally forward and downward from the lower borders of the first 11 ribs to the upper borders of the last 11 ribs, lifting the ribs upward and outward; the internal intercostals course downward and posteriorly from the inner surface of the ribs near the sternum to the upper border of the rib below, pulling the ribs downward and inward. Function during inhalation and exhalation.

Internal rotation. An inward turning of a limb toward the body.

Intrinsic tongue muscles. Four muscles within the tongue body that change the shape of the tongue, including the superior longitudinal, inferior longitudinal, transverse, and vertical muscles.

Inversion. A medial movement of the plantar surface of the foot, directing it toward midline.

Ischial tuberosities. Posterior portions of the base of the pelvis that serve as a weightbearing surface in sitting.

Jaw stabilization. Active, internal jaw control with minimal up/down jaw movements, especially significant in cupdrinking.

Kinesthesia. The sense perception of movement.

Labial. Pertaining to the lips.

Labyrinthine head righting. A postural reaction elicited by stimulation of the labyrinthine receptors in the middle ear that results in contraction of the neck muscles to orient the head in a vertical position.

Landau. A postural reaction in which the head elevates and the spine and limbs extend when the body is held horizontally suspended in the prone position; probably a combination of righting reactions.

Laryngopharynx. The part of the pharynx extending from the hyoid bone down to the laryngeal and esophageal openings.

Larynx. A valving system, starting at the base of the tongue and extending down to the top of the trachea, designed to keep food from entering the airway; structurally it consists of the epiglottis, valleculae, piriform sinuses, false vocal folds, true vocal folds, aryepiglottic folds, and the cuneiform, cricoid, thyroid, and arytenoid cartilages.

Lateral pinch. The object is held between the thumb and side of a curled index finger.

Lingual. Pertaining to the tongue.

Mandible. The lower jaw, consisting of the body with its alveolar processes and the ramus with its condyloid and coronoid processes.

Masseter muscle. The most powerful of the jaw muscles coursing from the zygomatic arch (cheekbone) to the angle and ramus of the mandible; assists in elevating the jaw for closure with slow, powerful contraction especially important during chewing.

Maxilla. The upper jaw that borders the oral cavity, nasal cavity, and orbits of the eyes; formed by alveolar and palatine processes.

Medial scapular muscles. Refers to trapezius and rhomboids.

Monocular vision. Vision in which the image from an inactive eye is ignored or suppressed by the central nervous system.

Munching. Early chewing activity composed of rhythmical up/down jaw movements with spreading, flattening, and some up/down tongue movements.

Nasopharynx. The part of the pharynx from the soft palate up to the base of the skull, including the opening to the nasal cavity.

Neck righting. A postural reaction, elicited by joint receptors of the neck, that results in the body and limbs aligning themselves with the head.

Non-reduplicated babbling. Variegated babbling consisting of long chains of different consonant-vowel combinations.

Oblique muscles. The external and internal muscles of the abdominal wall that connect the pelvis/hips to the ribs as they course up and outward and up and inward, respectively; they actively pull the ribs down and compress the abdominal wall during respiration; they functionally work together to flex, laterally flex, and rotate the trunk.

Oculomotor. Referring to muscles of the eye.

Optical righting. A postural reaction elicited by stimulation of visual receptors that results in an upright orientation of the head and body in relation to the environment.

Oral cavity. Area bounded superiorly by the hard and soft palates, posteriorly by the posterior faucial arch, laterally by the alveolar ridges and cheeks, anteriorly by the alveolar ridges and lips, inferiorly by the tongue and its soft tissue connection to the mandible.

Oral mechanism. Structurally composed of the maxilla, mandible, lips, cheeks, tongue, floor of the mouth, hard and soft palates, uvula, and anterior and posterior faucial arches, including corresponding musculature and soft tissue.

Orbicularis oris. Sphincter-like muscle of the lips involved in lip protrusion, rounding, and closure.

Oropharynx. The part of the pharynx that extends downward from the soft palate to the hyoid bone and is continuous with the oral cavity.

Palmar grasp. Occurs when an object is held with fingers flexed and thumb adducted. The distal digit of the thumb is often flexed.

Pectoralis major. The muscle that adducts and internally rotates the humerus. In addition, the clavicular portion flexes the humerus while the sternal portion extends the humerus from a flexed position.

Periodic breathing. Characterized by brief apneic periods or respiratory pauses of 3 seconds or greater that are interrupted by respirations of 20 seconds or less in duration.

Permanent teeth. The 32 secondary or adult teeth that begin to appear at approximately six years of age.

Pharyngeal cavity. Area bounded by the pharynx, which is a musculomembraneous tube that extends downward from the sphenoid bone at the base of the skull to the laryngeal and esophageal openings; it is subdivided into the nasopharynx, oropharynx, and laryngopharynx.

Pharyngeal mechanism. Primarily composed of the pharynx (see pharyngeal cavity), the three pharyngeal constrictors, the four internal longitudinal muscles of the pharyngeal wall, and the epiglottis and hyoid bone, including corresponding musculature and soft tissue.

Phonation. The generation of voiced sound.

Physiological flexion. Term used to describe the general tendency for flexion in the full-term newborn infant; mechanism is unknown, but results in recoil of flexed limbs when passively extended; provides stability for early posture and random movements.

Pincer grasp. Occurs when a pellet-sized object is held between the distal pads of the thumb and index finger.

Pinch. To hold a pellet-sized object between the tip of the finger and thumb.

Piriform sinuses. Recesses or depressions in the posterior laryngopharynx that are lateral to the cricoid and arytenoid cartilages and medial to the thyroid cartilage.

Plantar flexion. A movement of the foot away from the anterior aspect of the lower leg.

Postural accompaniments. Postural control strategies that occur immediately prior to and during movement; controlled by a feedforward mechanism.

Postural preparations. Postural control strategies that occur before movement to set a stable posture, including changing the base of support and muscle cocontraction patterns to stiffen joints; utilizes feedforward control.

Postural reactions. Feedback-type strategies of postural control that occur when balance is disturbed unexpectedly, primarily by an external source.

Primary standing. A newborn postural reaction that results in the baby standing upright when placed on the feet with the trunk supported.

Pronation. Occurs when the forearm is rotated so the palm of the hand points backward when the arm is in an anatomical position.

Proprioception. Stimulus originating in the muscles, tendons, and soft tissue.

Protective extension. A postural reaction resulting in straightening of the arms or legs toward a supporting surface in an attempt to stop a fall.

Quadriceps. Muscle group of the anterior thigh that extends the knee; the rectus femoris portion also can flex the hip.

Radial-digital grasp. To hold an object with an opposed thumb and fingertips. The space visible between the thumb and fingers indicate that the palmar arches are active.

Radial-palmar grasp. Occurs when the fingers press the object against the radial side of the hand and opposed thumb.

Raking. Using the fingers to draw small objects into the palm.

Rectus abdominus. The midline abdominal muscle that originates at the sternum and inserts on the pubis; its action produces flexion of the lower trunk and a backward tipping of the top of the pelvis.

Reduplicated babbling. Long chains of repeated consonant-vowel combinations.

Respiration. The exchange of oxygen and carbon dioxide between the atmosphere and the cells of the body through the process of inhalation (inspiration) and exhalation (expiration).

Rib cage. Structurally composed of the 12 ribs, sternum, thoracic vertebrae, and corresponding musculature and soft tissue attachments.

Rib flaring. Expansion of the lower ribs that occurs as the diaphragm contracts, pulling the ribs up and out on inhalation.

Righting reactions. Postural reactions that bring the head and trunk into an upright position in space.

Rooting response. A food-seeking movement in response to tactile input presented on the lips or cheeks, characterized by mouth opening and head turning in the direction of the touch; occurs until approximately four-five months of age.

Rotary jaw movements. Activity used in chewing that reflects the integration of up/down, forward/backward, diagonal, diagonal-rotary, and circular-rotary movements of the jaw.

Rotator cuff muscles. A large group of muscles that rotates the humerus and stabilizes it in the glenoid fossa.

Scapular abductors. A group of muscles that move the scapula away from the spine.

Scapular adductors. A group of muscles that move the scapula toward the spine.

Scapular downward rotation. Movement of the inferior border of the scapula toward the spine.

Scapular upward rotation. Movement of the inferior border of the scapula away from the spine.

Scapular winging. Separation of the scapula from the chest wall.

Scapulohumeral musculature. Referring to muscles that originate on the scapula and move the humerus.

Scapulothoracic musculature. Referring to muscles that originate on the thorax and move the scapula.

Serratus anterior. The muscle that originates on the upper eight ribs and inserts on the vertebral border of the scapula to protract and upwardly rotate the scapula. It also stabilizes the scapula against the chest wall.

Shoulder girdle depression. Movement of the shoulder toward the pelvis.

Shoulder girdle elevation. Movement of the shoulder toward the ear.

Soft palate. The velum or pharyngeal palate posterior to the hard palate composed of a median fibromuscular bundle and musculature attachments; raises and lowers to create velopharyngeal closure.

Sternoclavicular joint. Relating to the articulation between the sternum and the clavicle.

Sucking. A rhythmical method of obtaining liquid and food using small up/down jaw movements, up/down tongue movements, lip approximation, and cheek activity that creates negative pressure in the oral cavity.

Sucking pads. Round, encapsulated fatty tissue deposits within the cheeks of the young infant; buccal fat pads.

Suckling. An early lick-type of sucking pattern characterized by rhythmical forward/backward tongue movements, large rhythmical up/down and forward/backward jaw movements, and minimal cheek and lip activity.

Supination. A rotation of the forearm in which the palm is facing forward when the arm is in the anatomical position.

Suprahyoid muscles. A group of six muscles, including the digastric, mylohyoid, and geniohyoid muscles (jaw depressors), the hyoglossus and genioglossus muscles (extrinsic tongue muscles), and the stylohyoid muscle, that suspend the hyoid bone from the jaw and skull and move it forward, backward, and upward; with the infrahyoids, these muscles fix the hyoid in position and assist in head flexion.

Swallowing. The act of deglutition in which material is collected and moved from the mouth posteriorly through the pharynx and esophagus into the stomach.

Temporomandibular joint. The joint formed by the articulation of the superior condyloid process of the mandible and the zygomatic process of the temporal bone of the skull.

Three-jaw chuck. To hold an object with the thumb and first two fingers.

Tongue. The tongue body is composed of intrinsic tongue muscles, soft tissue, mucosal covering, and on its superior surface, the papillae and taste buds; primarily located in the oral cavity, its posterior aspect and extrinsic musculature also connect it with the pharyngeal cavity; described in terms of its tip, blade, dorsum, and root.

Tongue lateralization. Active movements of the tongue to the sides of the mouth to maintain and propel food between the biting surfaces during the chewing process.

Unilateral reach. The ability to reach with one arm.

Valleculae. Depressions bordered anteriorly by the base of the tongue, posteriorly by the epiglottis, and laterally by the pharyngeal walls.

Variegated babbling. See non-reduplicated babbling.

Velopharyngeal closure. Closing off of the nasal cavity from the oral and pharyngeal cavities through action of the soft palate and pharyngeal wall; occurs during swallowing and speech.

Ventilation. The process of exchange or movement of air between the lungs and room air.